INTERNAL MEDICINE WORDS

compiled by
Minta Oliver Danna, MT

edited by
Patricia Bowen, CMT

Rayve Productions

Senior Editor: Barbara F. Ray
Manuscript Editor: Pat Bowen, CMT
Research Editor: Serena Standley
Cover Design: Royal Windsor Graphics

Rayve Productions Inc.
Box 726 Windsor CA 95492 USA

Text copyright © 1997 Minta Oliver Danna

Printed in the United States of America

Publisher's Cataloging in Publication
Danna, Minta Oliver
  Internal medicine words / Minta Danna. — 1st ed.
  p. cm.
  Includes bibliographical references and index.
  ISBN 1-877810-68-1

  1. Internal medicine—Dictionaries.   2. Medicine—Dictionaries.
  3. Internal medicine—Terminology.   4. Medicine—Terminology.

  I. Title

RC41.D36 1997   610'.3
                       QBI97—40446
Library of Congress Catalog Card Number 97-065052

To Gil, Joe and Joy,
with love

Contents

About the Author

Minta Danna was born in Austin, Texas and, with her father in the Army, lived in a variety of locales. She attended thirteen different schools, the first in Germany and the last, Texas Christian University, in Fort Worth, Texas.

Her professional life has been varied, too, starting with teaching English in the District of Columbia. Later at the USDA Southern Regional Research Laboratory in New Orleans, she did scientific manuscript typing for many years before making an exciting change to teletypist at the New Orleans Lakefront Airport.

Then she discovered the fascinating world of medical transcription at Ochsner Clinic in New Orleans. Minta appreciated her new profession's standards of excellence, and she thrived on the daily challenges encountered while transcribing. Moreover, she found the process of learning new medical words great fun—not unlike working a crossword puzzle.

Minta Danna's fascination with words led her to begin collecting medical terms, and her three-column notebook grew quickly. Soon, copies were seen, open, on all the transcriptionists' desks, as they remain today, seven years later. Minta still makes new entries most every day, even as she realizes a dream come true—seeing her medical word list in book form.

Minta Danna is the mother of three adult children. She currently lives and works in New Orleans, Louisiana, and is a member of the American Association for Medical Transcription.

Acknowledgments

Completion of this book would not have been possible without the help of many medical transcriptionists and other talented professionals who contributed to the project.

From the author . . .
Thanks to Joanne F. McConnon, my medical transcription mentor at Ochsner, for the tough training and uncompromising commitment to excellence she imparted, which has served me well both in my career and in this endeavor.

I offer heartfelt thanks to my friends and fellow transcriptionists Connie Polsey, Gilda Barger, Janice Welman, Gwendolyn Harris, Barbara Daughdrill and Karen Brown. They lent their listening skills to find the words we were hearing, their research expertise, their own word lists and their unfailing support and encouragement to me in the preparation of this book.

And most of all, thanks to my publisher, Rayve Productions, for polishing and preparing my manuscript for publication, and for believing it will prove a useful addition to the field of Internal Medicine transcription.

From the publisher . . .
Special thanks to Pat Bowen, CMT, for so meticulously editing and proofing the manuscript, and for her many significant recommendations which improved the book.

Thanks, too, to Donna Avila-Weil, CMT and author, for reviewing the project and providing invaluable input regarding content and style.

Appreciation is also extended to Serena Standley, editor and researcher, and Martha A. Mathiews and her staff, cover design consultants.

Publisher's Preface

Medical transcriptionists frequently contact us to request or recommend that we publish specific new health language word books not currently in print. Although there are many excellent word books available, health language professionals are always eager for new, focused references that will aid in the accuracy and speed of their work.

To help meet the needs of those whose work focuses on internal medicine, we have published *Internal Medicine Words*. For more than seven years, medical transcriptionist Minta Danna gathered, compiled and edited this comprehensive internal medicine word list. A perfectionist (and what excellent medical transcriptionist isn't?), she passionately fine-tuned her word list each day.

Minta Danna shared her internal medicine word list with a few work associates, and soon, other transcriptionists were requesting it, too. Now, it is with great pleasure that we offer to you Minta Danna's expanded *Internal Medicine Words*.

Please note . . . The numerous definitions and brief descriptions included with Minta Danna's *Internal Medicine Words* are intended only as word aids to help speed transcription work. For precise, comprehensive definitions of medical terms, refer to one of the many authoritative medical dictionaries, encyclopedias, or other fine medical resources currently available.

Thank you for sharing our world of words, and when you discover a new word you would like Rayve Productions to include in the next edition of *Internal Medicine Words*, please contact us.

Explanatory Notes

Accuracy and Style
The internal medicine words in this book have been thoroughly reviewed for accuracy and, in recognition of generally accepted medical transcription professional standards, every attempt has been made to adhere to the style guidelines of the American Association for Medical Transcription (AAMT).

However, in the world of medical language, as in language generally, there are many variables in word and style, each of which may be accurate. In those instances where accuracy is not an issue, the final choice between variant spellings, or in the use of hyphens, possessives or other factors, is a matter of personal preference.

Alphabetical Organization and Cross-indexing
In this reference book, entries are alphabetized letter by letter as spelled, ignoring punctuation, spaces, prefixed numbers, or characters. Cross-indexing is extensive.

Hyphenation
Multiple eponyms are hyphenated. As explained above, this is a matter of personal style preference.

Possessives
Possessive forms have been dropped to conform to the guidelines of the American Association for Medical Transcription. Again, use of possessives is a matter of style preference.

Key Words, Synonyms and Explanatory Material
Word roots are in boldface type, e.g., **micro-**

Key words and phrases are in standard type and may be followed by a synonym, explanatory material, or both.

Synonyms are in standard type, separated from the key word by a virgule, a forward slash (/). For added clarification, a few synonyms felt to be less than obvious are noted "syn."

Explanatory material is in italic type, separated from the key word by a virgule, a forward slash (/).

Drugs — both generic and brand names — are in standard type.

Abbreviations
Abbreviations derived from foreign words or phrases are so designated (L., Latin; G., Greek), with the foreign words in italic type, followed by the English translation. For example:

> **q.h.** / L. *quaque hora* / every hour

Explanatory information and connecting words needed to expand an abbreviated term or phrase are in parentheses. For example:

> **NANB** / non-A, non-B (hepatitis)

> **SBE** / shortness (of) breath (on) exertion

Additional Information
Additional information following key words is not intended to be comprehensive, but to serve only as an aid to medical transcription. For comprehensive information regarding any medical term or drug, refer to one of the many authoritative medical dictionaries, encyclopedias, or other fine medical resources currently available.

Abbreviation Key
Drug — D
Over-the-counter drug — [OTC]
Test — T
Lab test — L
Latin — L.
Greek — G.

Selected References

Bennington, James L. *Encyclopedia and Dictionary of Laboratory Medicine.* Philadelphia: W. B. Saunders Co., 1984.

Bergey's Bacteria Words. Baltimore: Williams & Wilkins, 1992.

Dorland's Illustrated Medical Dictionary, 28th ed. Philadelphia: W. B. Saunders Co., 1994.

Cardiology Words and Phrases. Modesto: Health Professions Institute, 1995.

Drake, Ellen, and Randy Drake. *Saunders Pharmaceutical Word Book.* Philadelphia: W. B. Saunders Co., 1996.

Fordney, Marilyn and Marcy Diehl. *Medical Transcription Guide.* Philadelphia: W. B. Saunders Co., 1990.

Golish, Joseph A. *Diagnostic Procedure Handbook.* Baltimore: Williams & Wilkins, 1992.

Grant's Atlas of Anatomy, 9th ed. Baltimore: Williams & Wilkins, 1991.

Laboratory Test Handbook, 4th ed. Hudson: Lexi-Comp, 1996.

Lance, L.L. *Quick Look Drug Book.* Baltimore: Williams & Wilkins, 1996.

Lyons, Albert S. and R. Joseph Petrucelli, II. *Medicine, An Illustrated History.* New York: Abradale Press, 1987.

Orthopedic Words and Phrases. Modesto: Health Professions Institute, 1994.

Physician's Desk Reference (PDR), 51st ed. Montvale: Medical Economics Co., Inc., 1997.

Pyle, V. *Current Medical Terminology*, 5th ed. Modesto: Health Professions Institute, 1996.

Sloan, Sheila B. *A Word Book in Pathology and Laboratory Medicine.* Philadelphia: W. B. Saunders Co., 1984.

Sloan, Sheila B. *The Medical Word Book*, 3rd ed. Philadelphia: W. B. Saunders Co., 1982.

Stedman's Abbreviations, Acronyms & Symbols. Baltimore: Williams & Wilkins, 1992.

Stedman's GI/GU Words, 2nd ed. Baltimore: Williams & Wilkins, 1996.

Stedman's Medical Dictionary, 26th ed. Baltimore: Williams & Wilkins, 1995.

Stedman's Medical Speller, 2nd ed. Baltimore: Williams & Wilkins, 1995.

Webster's Medical Speller, 2nd ed. Springfield: Merriam-Webster Inc., 1995.

ALPHABETICAL LISTING

OF

INTERNAL MEDICINE WORDS

-a / (pl.) **-ae** / *a noun ending added to a root element*
  forms the name of a thing / e.g., derm**a**, gingiv**a**

A$_2$ / *hemoglobin*

AAS / aortic arch syndrome

Ab / abortion

abasia / *inability to walk*

abciximab / ReoPro / *prevents blood clot formation* / D

ABD / abdomen / abdominal

abdominis / *muscles*

abducens / abducent / abducting / *drawing away*

abduction / *abnormal movement/drift of body part*

abductor digiti minimi manus / *muscle of little finger*

abductor digiti quinti minimi / *muscles*

abductor digiti minimi pedis / *muscle of little toe*

abductor hallucis / *abductor muscle of great toe*

abductor ossis metatarsi quinti / *muscles*

abductor pollicis brevis / *muscle of thumb, short*

abductor pollicis longus / *muscle of thumb, long*

abductovalgus / adductovarus (Pod)

abetalipoproteinemia / *blood disorder*

ABGs / arterial blood gases

ablation / *detachment or removal*

abscess / *localized collection of pus*

Absorbine Jr. / *athlete's foot* / D [OTC]

-ac / *pertaining to* / *affected by* / e.g., mani**ac**

a.c. / L. *ante cibum* / before meals
  also ... p.c. / L. *post cibum* / after meals

AC / acromioclavicular / *shoulder*

acanthocyte / acanthrocyte / *cell*

acanthosis, nigricans / *epidermal thickening, as in psoriasis*

acapnia / *lack of carbon dioxide in the blood*

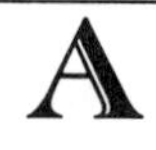

Additional Entries

____

____

____

____

acarbose / Precose / *drug study*
accelerator urinae / *muscles*
accessorius / *muscles*
Accolate / *for asthma* / D
accretio cordis (Cardio)
Accu-Chek / *for sugar* / T
Accupril / quinapril / D / *to regulate blood pressure*
Accutane / D / *for severe cystic acne*
ACE / angiotensin-converting enzyme / *inhibitors* / D
acebutolol (Vasc) / *antihypertensive* / D
acetabulum / acetabula (Ortho) / *depression on hip bone*
acetaminophen / *analgesic* / D
acetazolamide / *anticonvulsant* / D
acetylcholine / *vasodilator* / D
acetylcholinesterase / *enzyme*
Ace wrap / *for sprain, swelling*
achalasia / *failure to relax*
Achilles tendon / *heel*
achlorhydria / *no HCl*
acholic / *free from bile*
achondroplasia / *dwarfism*
achromasia / *absence of normal pigmentation*
Achromycin / *broad-spectrum antibiotic* / D
achylia / *absence of gastric juice or digestive secretions*
acid-fast cultures
acid hemolysin / T
acid phosphatase
acidophilus
acidosis / *decrease in pH*
Aci-Jel / *vaginal jelly* / D
acinar/-ization

Additional Entries

____

____

____

____

acini/-us / *small saclike dilatation*
acinic cell carcinoma
Acinetobacter
aclasia / *a breaking*
Aclovate / *topical anti-inflammatory* / D
acne conglobata (Derm) / *scarring*
acne rosacea (Derm)/ *flushing of nose, forehead and cheeks*
acne vulgaris (Derm) / *common acne*
acneiform eruption
acous- / acousti- / *hearing* / *sound* / e.g., **acoust**ical
acro- / *extremity* / *end* / *tip* / e.g., **acro**arthritis
acroarthritis / *inflammation of joints of the feet or hands*
acrochordon / skin tag / *small, pendulous growth on skin*
acrocyanosis / *circulatory disorder*
acrokeratosis (Derm) / *overgrowth of horny skin layer*
acromegaly / *enlargement of peripheral body parts*
acromial (Ortho)
acromioclavicular (Ortho)
acromion / *pertaining to the shoulder*
acropachy / *clubbing* / *bone changes*
acroparesthesia / *tingling of extremities*
acrosclerosis / *stiffness and tightness of skin of fingers*
ACS HTF guide wire (Cardio) / *in cardiac catheterization*
ACTH / adrenocorticotropic hormone
Acthar / *gel* / *steroid* / D
Actifed / *antihistamine* / D [OTC]
Actigall / *gallstone dissolving agent* / D
actinic keratoses (Derm) / *yellow or brown marginated lesions on elderly skin* / *from sun exposure*
Actinomyces / *bacteria*
actinomycin d / *antibiotic antineoplastic* / D

Additional Entries

____
____
____
____

Acular / D
acuminatum / *pointed*
acus-, acous- / *sound* / e.g., **acus**is, **acous**tic
acusis / normal hearing
acyclovir / Zovirax / *for herpes* / D
acylcarnitine / *amino acid*
ad- *toward* / e.g., cephal**ad**, **ad**nerval, **ad**axial
a.d. / L. *ad libitum* / *as desired*
Adalat / *antianginal* / D
adamantinoma / *a rare tumor, usually occurring in the tibia*
Adams-Stokes (Cardio)
Adapin / *antidepressant* / D
adaptic
adaptive scale
ADD / attention deficit disorder
Addis count / *cells*
adduct / *toward midline*
adductor hallucis / *adductor muscle of great toe*
adductor longus / magnus / minimus / pollicis / *muscles*
adductus primus varus / *bowlegged*
ADEKs / *chewable vitamin supplement* / D
aden- / *gland* / *sweat* / e.g., **aden**oma
adenocarcinoma (Onc) / *cancer derived from glandular tissue*
Adenocard / *injection*
adenoma / *tumor cells that form glands or glandlike structures*
adenomatous
adenomyosis
adenopathies / *enlargement of the glands, especially lymph glands*
adenosine thallium study / T
adenovillous
ADH / antidiuretic hormone (vasopressin)

Additional Entries
____
____
____
____

ADHD / attention deficit hyperactivity disorder
adherence/-ent
adiadochokinesia / *inability to perform rapidly alternating movements*
Adie pupil
adip-, adipo- / *fat* / *fatty* / e.g., **adip**osity
adipose / *fatty*
adjuvant / *substance added to drug that affects active ingredient*
ad lib / L. *ad libitum* / as desired
ADLs / activities of daily living
adnexa (both singular and plural) / (L. connected parts) / *connections* / *ties* / e.g., a. oculi / *lacrimal glands*; a. uteri / *ovaries and oviducts*
adnexa and fundus
Adrenalin 1:1000/ml
adrenergic receptor / *epinephrine*
Adriamycin / *antibiotic antineoplastic* / D
Adson maneuver / *neck, for thoracic outlet syndrome*
adult onset asthma
adventitia/-ial
aegis / *protecting influence* / *power*
aer- / **aero-** / *air* / *atmosphere* / e.g., **aer**ate, **aer**ial
aerobe / *an organism requiring oxygen to live* / e.g., bacterium
AeroBid inhaler / *for asthma* / D
AeroChamber / *inhaler*
aerodontalgia / *pain in teeth*
Aeromonas shigelloides / *bacteria*
aerophagia / *to swallow air*
aeruginosa (Pseudomonas)
AFB / acid fast bacilli / *smear*

Additional Entries

____

____

____

____

afebrile / *without fever*
afferent / *fluid or nerve impulses flowing* **inward**
   (opposite) efferent / *fluid or nerve impulses flowing* **outward**
Afrin / *nasal spray* / D
aflatoxin / Aspergillus flavus toxin / *most potent known carcinogen*
AFO / ankle foot orthosis
AG / albumin-globulin ratio
agammaglobulinemia
aganglionic / *characterized by the absence of ganglion cells*
agenesis / *not developed*
agglutinin / *antibody*
Agiolax / *laxative*
agitator caudae / *muscles*
Aggrastat (experimental) / tirofiban / *glycoprotein blocker in*
   unstable angina / *prevents blood clot formation* / D
aggravated
aggregometer / *instrument for measuring platelet adhesiveness*
agnogenic / *unknown etiology*
agnosia / *inability to comprehend*
agonist / *drug activator*
AI / aortic insufficiency
AIDS / acquired immune deficiency syndrome
Aircast
air contrast barium enema
air splint
Air stirrup brace (Ortho)
AKA / above knee amputation / also known as
akathisia / *inability to sit still*
Akcoline / D
akinesia/-etic / *loss of motor function*
Akin's, Dr. / *mouthwash*

Additional Entries

____

____

____

____

-al / *pertaining to* / e.g., vert**al**, method**al**, abdomin**al**

ALA mg, 24hr

ala nasi / *outer side of nose*

Albalon (Oph) / *solution*

albicans / *white*

Albright syndrome

albumin / *simple protein*

albuminuria / proteinuria / *protein in urine*

albuterol / Ventolin inhaler / D

Aldactazide / *diuretic* / *antihypertensive* / D

Aldactone / *potassium sparing diuretic* / D

Aldomet / *antihypertensive* / D

Aldoril / *antihypertensive* / D

aldolase levels

aldosterone / *hormone* / D

aldosteronism / *excessive secretion of hormone aldosterone*

Aldrich-Wiskott syndrome

Alendronate / Fosamax / *for bone strengthening* / *for osteoporosis* / D

Aleve / Naprosyn / *nonsteroidal* / D

-alge-, algesi-, algia-, algio-, algo- / *pain* / *sensitivity to pain* /
  e. g., an**alge**sic, neur**algia**

alginolyticus / *bacteria*

aliquot / *evenly dividing number*

alkaline phosphatase

alkalinization

alkalosis / alkalotic / *abnormally high alkalinity of body fluids*

Alka-Seltzer / *analgesic* / D

Alkeran / *antineoplastic* / D

alkylate/-ing / *therapy*

Allegra / *nonsedating antihistamine* / *for allergies* / D

Allen test / *glucose in urine* / T

Additional Entries

____

____

____

____

allergen / *anything that induces a state of allergy*
allergosorbent / T
allograft / *graft of tissue—same species*
allopurinol / Zyloprim / *for gout* / D
ALS / amyotrophic lateral sclerosis
alopecia areata (Derm) / *scalp* / *hair loss*
alpha$_1$-antichymotrypsin
alpha$_1$-antitrypsin
alpha-fetoprotein
alpha interferon
Alport syndrome / *in the deaf, congenital glomerulonephritis*
alprazolam / Xanax / *antianxiety agent* / D
alprostadil / *vasodilator* / D
ALT (SGPT) / Alanine Aminotransferase
Altace / *antihypertensive* / D
Altemeier / *surgical procedure*
alteplase, recombinant / t-pa / TPA / tissue plasminogen activator /
    blood clot dissolver / D
ALTernaGEL / *antacid* / D
Alternaria / *allergen*
altram...**NO!** (see "Ultram")
Alupent inhaler / D
alveolar / *pertaining to an alveolus, a small, saclike dilatation*
alveolus/-eoli (pl.) / *air cells in the lungs*
Alzheimer disease / *dementia*
amantadine / *antiparkinsonian* / D
amaurosis fugax / *momentary blindness*
ambi-, ambo- / *on both sides* / e.g., **ambi**dextrous
ambilateral / *pertaining to both sides*
amblyopia / *decreased vision*
Ambien / *sedative* / D

Additional Entries

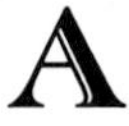

ameb- / *change* / *a protozoan that constantly changes its shape* / e.g., **ameb**a, **amoeb**a
amebiasis / *infestation with amoebas, especially parasites in the intestines*
amel- / *enamel* / e.g., en**amel**oblastoma
Amen / *for abnormal uterine bleeding* / D
amenorrhea / *absence of menses*
ametropia (Oph)
AMI / acute myocardial infarction
Amicar / aminocaproic acid / *hemostatic agent* / D
amikacin / *antibacterial* / D
amiloride / *potassium-sparing diuretic* / D
aminocaproic acid / Amicar / *systemic hemostatic* / *to control excessive bleeding* / D
aminoglutethimide / Cytadren / *antineoplastic* / D
aminoguanidine / *for diabetes* / D
aminophylline / *bronchodilator* / D
amiodarone / *antiarrhythmic* / D
amitriptyline / *antidepressant* / D
amlodipine / *calcium channel blocker* / D
amnion / *embryonic membrane*
amorphous / *without definite shape*
amoxapine / *antidepressant* / *D*
amoxicillin / *antibiotic* / D
Amoxil / *penicillin-type antibiotic* / D
Amphojel / *antacid* / D [OTC]
amphoric / *breathing*
amphotericin B / *antifungal* / D
amphi-, **ampho-** / *both* / *on both sides* / *in two ways* / *around* / e.g., **amphi**bian, **amphi**theater
ampicillin / *antibiotic* / D

Additional Entries

ampulla of Vater / hepatopancreatica
amrinone / Inocor / *cardiotonic* / *for congestive heart failure* / D
amyl- , amylo- / *starch* / e.g., **amyl**ase
amylase/-ase / *enzymes that help convert starch to sugar*
amylasuria
amyloid/-osis
amyopathic dermatomyositis
amyotrophy/-ic / *muscle wasting*
an-, a- / *without* / *not* / e.g., **an**aerobic
ANA / antinuclear antibodies / *profile*
ANA 1:640 (*when titer, use colon*)
anabolic / *promoting conversion into living matter*
Anadrol / *steroid for anemias* / D
anaerobic / *lacking molecular oxygen*
anaerococcus
Anafranil / *for obsessive compulsive disorders* / D
anagrelide / *antithrombotic* / D
analgesics / *compounds that relieve pain*
Analpram-HC / *anorectal cream* / D
anal verge
anaphylactoid / *resembling anaphylaxis*
anaphylaxis / *decreased resistance to a toxin*
anaplasia / *decrease in structural differentiation*
Anaprox / *nonsteroidal anti-inflammatory* / D
anasarca / *edema fluid filtering into subcutaneous tissue*
Anaspaz / *antispasmodic* / D
anastomosis / *a connection between two vessels*
anatomic / *structure of organism*
ANCA / anti-neutrophil cytoplasmic antibody (testing) / T
Ancef / *injection* / *antibiotic* / D
anconeus / *muscle* / *elbow*

Additional Entries

andr-, **andro-** / *male* / *masculine* / e.g., **andro**gen
androgen / *hormone that determines masculine charac-*
  teristics
androgenic / *masculine*
Android-10 / *androgen* / D
androstanediol / *androgen*
androstenediol / *androgen*
androstenedione / *an androgenic steroid produced by the*
  testes, adrenal cortex and ovary which can be converted
  metabolically to testosterone and other androgens
anemia / *iron deficiency* / e.g., hypochromic microcytic a.;
  macrocytic a.; sideroblastic a.
anergy / *lack of energy* / *lack of normal response to*
  substances
aneroid device / *for taking blood pressure*
aneurysm/ *abnormal balloonlike dilatation of a blood vessel*
aneurysmectomy / *surgical removal of the sac of an aneurysm*
ANF / antinuclear factor
angi-, **angio-** / *pertaining to blood vessels* /
  e.g., **angio**gram
angin- / *a choking* / *strangling* / e.g., **angin**a
angina pectoris (Cardio)
angioedema / *vascular*
angiography / *radiography of vessels injected with radiopaque*
  matter
angioma / *vascular swelling or tumor*
angiomata
angiotensin / *hormone*
angle of mandible
anhedonia / *inability to enjoy normal pleasures*
anhydrase / *an enzyme*

Additional Entries

____

____

____

____

anicteric/-sclera(e)
anion gap / *pertaining to ions*
aniso- / *not equal* / *dissimilar* / e.g., **aniso**metropia
anisocoria (Oph)
anisocytosis (Hemo)
anisometropia (Oph) / *difference in refractive power of the two eyes*
anisopoikilo/-cytosis
ankylo- / *bent* / *crooked* / *stiff* / *fused* / e.g., **ankylo**glossia
ankylobrachial
ankyloglossia / *fusion of the tongue to the floor of the mouth*
ankylosing hyperostosis
ankylosing spondylosis
anlage/-en (pl.) (Psych)
annular / anular (L. *annulus* / ring) / *circular* / *ring-shaped*
annuloplasty (Cardio)
annulus/-uli / *ring-shaped structure* / *ring-shaped*
anodmia / anosmia / *loss of sense of smell*
Anodynos / *analgesic* / *anti-inflammatory* / D
anomia / *inability to name objects*
anopsia (Oph)
anorectal / *pertaining to the anus and the rectum*
anorexia / *diminished appetite*
anorgasmy / *absence of orgasms*
anoscopy / *speculum exam of anus*
anosmia / *loss of sense of smell*
anovulatory / anovular / *absence of discharge of ovum*
anoxic/-emic / *extreme lack of oxygen in blood*
Ansaid / *nonsteroidal anti-inflammatory* / D
anserine / *inflammation of bursa, thigh and leg* / *characteristic of or resembling a goose*

Additional Entries

____

____

____

____

Anspor / D
Antabuse / *deters alcohol consumption* / D
antalgic / *gait shows pain*
ante- / *before*
antebrachial (Ortho) / *pertaining to the forearm*
antecubital (Ortho) / *pertaining to the elbow*
anteflexed / *to bend forward*
antegrade flow / *in the normal direction*
antergy / *resistance*
anterior cervical lymph nodes
antero- / *before*
anteroapical / *in front of an apex*
anterolateral / *situated in front and to one side*
anteroseptal / *in front of the septum of the heart*
anti- / *against*
anticardiolipin / *antibody study*
anticentromere / *chromosomes*
anticholinergic tricyclics / D
anticoagulated
anticollagen
anticonvulsant
anticus / anterior
antidepressant
antidiphosphopyridine nucleotidase
antigen / *substance that can stimulate an immune response*
antihistamine / *drug that opposes the action of a histamine* / D
antihistaminics
antimicrobial
antimitochondrial antibody
antineoplastic (Chemo)
antineural antibody

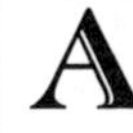

Additional Entries

antiphospholipid
antipyretic/-s
antiserum / (pl.) antisera / *serum that contains antibodies*
antiragicus / *muscles*
antistriational
antithrombocyte
antitrypsin / *a plasma protein produced in the liver*
Antivert / 25 mg / tab / *motion sickness preventative* / D
antr- / *cavity*, e.g., **antr**um
antra / *plural of antrum*
antral gastritis / antral erosions
antritis, maxillary / *inflammation of the antrum*
antrum / (pl.) antra / *any nearly closed cavity, especially in a bone*
-ant / *pertaining to* / *having characteristics of* / e.g., malign**ant**
Anturane / *for gout* / D
anucleated / *deprived of the nucleus*
anuria / anuric / *kidney shutdown*
Anusol-HC / *suppository cream*
-an, -ian / *belonging to* / *associated with* / e.g., Europ**ean**
anxiolytic / *antianxiety agent* / D
AO screw (Ortho)
aortic root
aortic SEM / (aortic) systolic ejection murmur
aortocoronary bypass
aortoiliac / *both the aorta and the iliac arteries*
A&P / anterior and posterior
   also ... auscultation and palpation / auscultation and percussion
a panic / *excessively high lab result*
apap / APAP / acetaminophen / Tylenol / D [OTC]
apatite / *generic name for some minerals including calcium*
aperistalsis / *absence of peristalsis*

Additional Entries

____

____

____

____

apex / *the extremity of a conical or pyramidal structure, such as the heart or the lung*

aphagia/-ic / *difficulty swallowing*

aphakia/-ic (Oph) / *absence of eye lens*

aphasia / aphrasia / *inability to speak*

aphthous / *ulcer*

apical / *at the apex*

aplastic anemia / *anemia that is unresponsive to therapy*

AP & Lat / anteroposterior and lateral

Apley compression maneuver

apo- / *deprived of* / *separated from* / e.g., **apo**dia

apodia / *congenital absence of feet*

aponeurosis/-itis

apoLipoproteinE / *apoE, apoE-4*

apophyseal / *joint*

apophysis/-sitis / *bony outgrowth*

appendiceal / *pertaining to an appendix*

apperception / *perception and interpretation of sensory stimuli*

applanation tonometries (Oph) / *flattening of cornea by pressure*

apraxia / *inability to coordinate body movements, for reasons other than motor or sensory impairment*

Apresazide / *antihypertensive* / *vasodilator* / D

Apresoline / *antihypertensive* / *vasodilator* / D

APTX / acute parathyroidectomy

Aquaglide astringent (Derm)

AquaMEPHYTON 10 mg/ml / *coagulant*

A quadratus lumborum

aqueductal stenosis

-ar / *pertaining to (words ending in -l or -le, in the form -ular)* / e.g., cir**cle**, cir**cular**

ara-C / cytarabine hydrochloride (Chemo) / D

Additional Entries

____

____

____

____

arachnid / Arachnida / *arthropods such as spiders, scorpions, mites, ticks*

arachnodactyly / *thin fingers and toes*

arachnoiditis (Neuro) / *inflammation of arachnoid membrane*

arachnophobia / arachnephobia / *morbid fear of spiders*

arcade of Frohse

arcus (L. a bow) / *structure having curved outline / resembling a bent bow or an arch / arc-shaped*

arcus corneae (Oph)

arcus lipoidalis (Oph)

arcus senilis (Oph)

areata (Derm) / *occurring in patches or a limited area / e.g., alopecia areata*

Aredia IV / *bone resorption suppressant* / D

areola / (pl.) areolae / (adj.) areolar / *small ring of color, as about the nipple of the breast*

ARF / acute respiratory failure

Argyll Robertson pupils

argon laser photocoagulation

Aristocort / triamcinolone / *topical corticosteroid* / D

Aristospan / *injectable replacement therapy in adrenocortical deficiency states* / D

Arliden / *for vertigo* / D

armamentarium / *all therapeutic means available*

Armour Thyroid / *for hypothyroidism* / D

Arnold-Chiari malformation (Neuro)

arrectores pilorum / *muscles*

arrhythmia / *loss of rhythm*

Artane / *antiparkinsonian* / D

arter-, arterio- / *pertaining to an artery* / e.g., **arterio**graphy

arteriography / *x-ray of arteries with dye*

Additional Entries

---

arteriolar
arteriole / *minute arterial branch*
arteriosclerosis obliterans
arteriovenous
arteritis, temporal
arthr-, arthro- / *joint* / *where bones meet* / e.g., **arthr**itis
arthralgia / *joint pain*
arthritides / *plural of arthritis*
arthritis / *inflammation in joint*
arthrocentesis / *aspiration of fluid from joint*
arthrodesis / *stiffening of joint as a result of surgery*
arthrogram / *x-ray of joint using dye*
arthrogryposis / *contraction of joint*
arthroplasties / *plastic surgeries of a joint*
arthroscopic
arthroscopy /(pronounced "ar-**thros**-copy") / *examination of the interior of a joint by means of an arthroscope*
articular / *pertaining to a joint*
articularis cubiti / genu / *muscles* / *triceps of the arm*
-ary / *pertaining to* / *connected with* / e.g., honor**ary**
aryepiglottic fold
aryepiglotticus muscle
arytenoid / *muscles*
ASA / acetylsalicylic acid / *aspirin* / D
Asacol (GI) / *for ulcerative colitis* / D
ASAP / as soon as possible (*less urgent than STAT or NOW*)
Ascaris lumbricoides or strongyloides / ascariasis / *roundworms*
Ascholl syndrome
ascites / (pronounced "as-**eye**-tees") / *accumulation of serous fluid in the peritoneal cavity*
Ascriptin / *buffered aspirin* / D [OTC]

Additional Entries

____
____
____
____

ascus, (pl.)asci / *spore case, lichens or fungi, consisting of a single terminal cell*
ASCVD / arteriosclerotic cardiovascular disease
ASD / atrial septal defect
-ase / *denotes an enzyme* / e.g., lip**ase**
asebic
Asendin / *antidepressant* / D
ASH / asymmetric septal hypertrophy
ASHD / arteriosclerotic heart disease
Asherman syndrome (Gyn)
-asis / *condition or state* / e.g., amebi**asis**
ASIS (Ortho) / anterior superior iliac spine
ASO titer / antistreptolysin-O (titer)
Aspercreme / *topical analgesic* / D
aspergillosis
aspergillus flavus / "aflatoxin" / *carcinogen*
asphyxia / *insufficient intake of oxygen*
asplenic / *absence of a spleen*
AST / Aspartate Aminotransferase
asteatosis / *diminished secretion of sebaceous glands*
asteatotic / *having eczema*
astemizole / Hismanal / *for seasonal allergic rhinitis* / D
astereognosis / *inability to recognize by touch*
asterion / *part of the skull*
asterixis / *motor disturbance*
asthenia / *without strength*
asthenic / *weak*
   (opposite) sthenic / *strong*
astr-, astra-, astro- / *star* / *star-shaped* / e.g., **astro**nomy
astragaloscaphoid joint
astragalus / *ankle bone*

Additional Entries

____
____
____
____

asymmetry / asymmetric
asystole (Cardio) / *no heart contractions / cardiac standstill*
Atarax / *anxiolytic* / D
ataxia / *inability to coordinate muscles*
atelectasis/-atic (Pulm) / *obstruction that keeps air out of part of the lung*
atenolol (Vasc) / *antiadrenergic* / D
-ate / *bring about / perform* / e.g., communi**cate**
atherectomy / *surgical removal of an atheroma in an artery*
atherogenesis / *formation of an atheroma*
atheroma / *lipid deposits in arteries*
atheromatous
atherosclerosis/-otic
athetotic/-oid/-osis / *slow, writhing involuntary movements*
-ation, -tion / *process* / e.g., decor**ation**
Ativan / *anxiolytic* / D
atlantoaxial (Ortho) / *joint between first two cervical vertebrae*
ATM / abnormal tubular myelin / *in cardiac cath reports*
atonic / *lacking normal tone or tension*
atonic bladder (Uro)
atopic dermatitis (Derm)
a torus palatinus (ENT) / *bony protuberance of hard palate*
atresia / *closed orifice* / e.g., biliary a.; aortic a.; bronchial a.; esophageal a.
Atrohist L.A. / *antihistamine / decongestant* / D
Atromid / *for cholesterol lowering* / D
atrophic / *wasting away*
atrophoderma of Pasini and Pierini
atrophozoites
atrophy / waste away

Additional Entries

____

____

____

____

atropine / *anticholinergic* / D
Atrovent inhalers / *bronchodilators* /D
attenuation / *thinning* / *weakening*
attrition / *rubbing away* / *wearing down* / *gradual diminution*
atypia / *not typical*
audiometry (Oto) / *testing of hearing*
Auerbach plexus
Aufranc-Turner / *operation*
Augmentin / penicillin-type antibiotic / D
aur- (Oto) / *the ear* / e.g., **aur**icular
Auralgan drops (Oto) / *analgesic* / D
aural glomus (Oto)
auricular (Oto)
Aurum Analgesic Cream / D
auscultation / *listening to sounds made by body structures*
auscultatory
Austin Flint (Cardio)
Austin Moore / *prosthesis*
auto- / *self* / *same one* / *self-caused* / e.g., **auto**immune
autoimmune / *arising from and directed against one's own tissues*
autoimmune hemolytic anemias
autoinsufflation
autologous / *self* / *own blood*
autosomal/-ly
AV dissociation (Cardio) / atrioventricular (dissociation)
AV fistula (Cardio) / atrioventricular (fistula)
A/V ratio (Oph) / arterio-venous (ratio)
avascular necrosis
AVC cream / sulfanilamide / *vaginal bacteriostatic* / D
Aveeno / *bath* / *moisturizer* / D
Aventyl / nortriptyline / *tricyclic antidepressant* / D

Additional Entries

____

____

____

____

avoidance reflex
avulsion / avulsed / *tearing away*
axial
Axid / nizatidine / *ulcer treatment* / D
axilla/-ae / *armpit*
axillary adenopathy / *swollen gland*
axis X- (Oph)
axonal / *axis of the body*
Axsain Cream / renamed Zostrix in 1992 / D
Aygestin / norethindrone / *for amenorrhea* D
azithromycin / Zithromax / *antibiotic* / D
Azlin / D
Azmacort inhaler / D
Azo Gantrisin / D
Azo-Standard / *urinary analgesic* / D [OTC]
azotemia / uremia (Uro) / e.g., nonrenal a. / prerenal a.
aztreonam / Azactam / *antibiotic* / D
Azulfidine / sulfasalazine / *for ulcerative colitis* / D
azurophil (Hemo)
azygous / *unpaired anatomical structure*

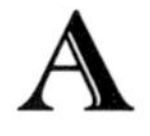

Additional Entries

____

____

____

____

B₁₂ / *vitamin*

B_{12} / *vitamin*
Babinski / *reflex*
bacitracin / *bacterial antibiotic* / D
baclofen / Lioresal / *muscle relaxant* / *antispastic* / D
bacteremia
Bacteroides fragilis
bacteruria / bacteriuria
Bactrim / *antibacterial* / *for urinary tract infections* / D
Bactroban / mupirocin / *antibiotic* / *for impetigo* / D
bagassosis / *respiratory disorder from sugar cane waste*
Bailey-Pignet (Ortho) / *bone age test* / T
baja patella / *below patella* / *low riding*
Baker cyst / *behind knee*
balanitis / *inflammation of glans penis*
ballistic exercise jerking
ballottable
ballottement / *palpatory technique to detect or examine a floating
    object in the body, such as an organ or fetus*
Balneol / *cream* / *for perianal cleansing* / D
Bancroft / *a parasitic disease*
Band-Aid
Bankart / *lesion of shoulder*
Bárány / Nylen-Bárány maneuver (Oto)
barbecue
Bardex / *bulb* / *catheter*
bariatric / *nutrition*
baritosis / *pneumonia due to inhalation of barium dust*
barium
Barlow syndrome (Cardio) / *mitral valve prolapse*
barotrauma (Oto) / *injury caused by pressure* / *in ear drum*
Barrett esophagus / *ulcer*

Additional Entries

____

____

____

____

Bartholin cyst (GYN) / *vaginal*
Bartonella/-osis / *cat scratch fever*
Bartter's syndrome / *hypokalemic alkalosis*
Basaljel / *antacid* / D
basal age / *highest mental age level of the Stanford-Binet intelli-
    gence scale at which all items are passed*
basilar crackles (Pulm) / *in lungs*
basilic vein / *vein in hand and forearm*
basophil / *a cell with granules that stain with basic dyes*
Bassini repair / *hernia*
Battey avian swine / *tuberculosis strain*
BCNU / BiCNU / bischloroethyl / *antineoplastic* / D
BE / barium enema
Beano / *for gas* / D
beats of clonus / *type of rapid muscle contractions*
Bechet disease (Gyn)
Bekhterev (Pod) / *reflex*
beclomethasone nasal inhaler / *Vanceril* / D
Beclovent oral inhaler / D
Beconase / *nasal inhaler* / D
Behcet syndrome (Derm)
Beelith / *dietary supplement* / D
beeturia / *pink to deep red colored urine after eating beets*
beignets
Beijing, China
Bekesky test (Oto) / *auditory test* / T
Bel-phen-ergot / *sedative* / *analgesic* / D
Bell-Horn knee sleeve
Bell palsy / *facial paralysis, usually temporary*
Bellergal-S / *sedative* / *analgesic* / D
Benadryl / *antihistamine* / D

Additional Entries

____
____
____
____

benazepril hydrochloride / Lotensin / *antihypertensive*
  (ACE inhibitor) / D
benefited
Benemid / probenecid / D
benign / *mild / not cancerous*
Bentyl / *gastrointestinal antispasmodic* / D
Benzagel / *for acne* / D
Benzamycin / *for acne* / D
benzathine penicillin G / D
benzodiazepines / *tranquilizers* / D
benzoyl peroxide / *keratolytic* / D
benztropine / *antiparkinsonian* / D
Bernoulli law / *trial*
Berocca Plus tabs / *vitamin mineral supplement* / D
berry aneurysm
beryllium / *metallic element*
beta-amyloid
beta blocker
Betagen / *antimicrobial surgical scrub* / D
Betagen Liquifilm / *eye drops* / D
Betadine / *antimicrobial* / D
Beta HCG screen / *pregnancy test* / T
betamethasone valerate cream / *corticosteroid* / D
Betapace (Cardio) / *antiarrhythmic* / D
betathalassemia minor / *anemia*
betaxolol / *antihypertensive beta blocker* / D
bethanechol / *urinary stimulant* / D
Betoptic (Oph) / *antiglaucomal* / D
bezoar / *concretion of hair or fibers found in stomach*
Biaxin / clarithromycin / *antibiotic* / D
Bicillin IM / *antibiotic* / D

B

Additional Entries

____
____
____
____

bicipital / *two heads* / *pertaining to biceps muscle*
bicornuate / *having two horn-shaped branches, as the uterus*
bicuspid aortic valve (Cardio)
b.i.d. / L. *bis in die* / *twice a day*
bifid / *split* / *separated into two parts*
bifida, spina
bifrontal
bifurcation / *division into two branches*
bigeminy / *pairing, especially heart beats in pairs*
bi-iliac bypass
bilateral foraminal stenosis
bilateral lateral
bile acid secretory diarrhea
bile acid sequestrant
bili- / *bile* / e.g., **bili**rubin
biliary atresia / *absence of major bile ducts*
biliary radicles
biliptysis / *bile in the sputum*
bilirubin / *red-yellow pigment in bile, urine, gallstones and blood*
Billroth disease (GI)
bin- / *two* / *both* / e.g., **bin**ary
Binswanger disease / *dementia*
bio- / *life* / e.g., **bio**graphy
bioavailability
bioptome / *cutting instrument for taking biopsy specimen*
Biofeet inserts / *used in shoes*
Bion Tears
biotinidase / *enzyme*
BiPAP / *used for sleep apnea* / *apparatus for O_2 delivery*
bipartite / *two parts*
bisferiens, pulsus / *striking twice*

Additional Entries

____

____

____

____

bismuth, milk of
bitemporal / *both temples or temporal bones*
Bjerrum scotoma (Oph)
Bjork-Shiley valve
BKA / below knee amputation
Blackfan-Diamond...**NO!**(seeDiamond-Blackfan syndrome)
Blalock-Taussig procedure
-blast, blasto- / *bud* / *sprout* / *embryonic cell*
blastocyst / blastocystic / *stage in embryo development*
Blastomyces/-in / *yeast*
bleb / bulla / *a large vesicle containing fluid*
bleomycin / Blenoxane (Onc) / *antineoplastic* / D
Blephamide (Oph) / *anti-inflammatory* / *eye drops* / D
blephar- / *eyelid*
blepharitis (Oph)
blepharophimosis (Oph)
blepharoplasty (Oph)
Blocadren / *migraine preventative* / D
Blom-Singer / *ossicular prosthesis* / *voice*
blood flow obstruction
blood gases: pCO_2 pO_2
Blount disease (Ortho)
blue dome cyst
blue nevus
BM / bowel movement
BMD / bone mineral density / T
Bochdalek / *diaphragmatic hernia*
Boeck sarcoid
Bohler angle
Bolvidon / *antidepressant* / D
bone island

Additional Entries

____

____

____

____

Bonfiglio graft (Ortho)
Bonine / meclizine hydrochloride / *for seasickness* / D [OTC]
borborygmus/ (pl.) -mi / *bowel sounds*
boss / bossing, frontal / (Fr. a swelling) / *rounded eminence, as on the surface of bone or tumor*
bosselated
Botox / botulinum toxin type A (Oph) / *for blepharospasm* / D
botryoid / *resembling a bunch of grapes*
Bouchard / *nodes*
bougie / *instrument used for dilating tubular organs*
BOW (Gyn) / bag of waters
BP / blood pressure
BPH / benign prostatic hypertrophy
Braasch / *catheter*
brachio- / *arm* / *radial*
brachiocephalic / *pertaining to both arm and head*
brachioplexus
brachioradialis / *muscles* / *forearm*
brachium / (pl.) brachia / *anatomical structure resembling an arm*
brachy- / *short* / e.g., **brachy**cephalic
brachy therapy (Onc)
brachycephalic / *abnormal shortness of head*
brady- / *slow* / *abnormal* / e.g., **brady**cardia
bradyarrhythmia / *abnormally slow heart rhythm*
bradycardia (Cardio) / *sinus* / *abnormally slow heartbeat*
bradykinesia/-etic / *decrease in movement*
bradykinin / *vasodilator*
Branhamella catarrhalis / *bacteria*
brash / water brash / *heartburn*
BRAT diet / bananas, rice cereal, applesauce and toast (diet)
Braxen / D

Additional Entries

____

____

____

____

brawny edema
BRCA1 / BRCA2 / *genes* / *associated with breast and
    ovarian cancer preventive surgery*
breast, shifting attenuation
Brethaire inhaler / D
Brethine / D
Brevicon / *oral contraceptive* / D
Bricanyl / *bronchodilator* / D
Brill-Symmers / *lymphoma*
Briquet hysteria / *somatization disorder* / *neurotic disorder*
Bristachol / Spanish Pravachol
Bristow procedure / *shoulder*
Broca (Neuro)
Bromfed / Bromfed-PD / *antihistamine* / D
bromocriptine / Parlodel / *antiparkinsonian* / D
brompheniramine / *antihistamine* / D
bronch- / *bronchus*
bronchi (Pulm) / *major branches from trachea to lungs*
bronchiectasis
bronchiolitis / bronchopneumonia
bronchoalveolar
bronchodilators
bronchopneumonia
bronchopulmonary
bronchoscopy
Bronkaid mist / *bronchodilator* / *D*
Bronkosol / *bronchodilator* / D
Brontex / *narcotic antitussive* / D
Brown-Buerger / *cystoscope sound*
Bruce protocol (Cardio)
Brown-Sequard (Neuro) / syndrome

B

Additional Entries

Brucella suis / *coccobacilli causing Brucellosis*
Brudzinski sign / *in neck* / *in meningitis*
bruits / *abnormal pulse sounds*
Brunner glands (GI)
Bruton / agammaglobulinemia
bruxism / *to grind teeth*
BSE / bilateral, symmetrical, equal
BSE pamphlet
BSER (Audiometry) / brainstem evoked response
BSO (Gyn) / bilateral salpingo-oophorectomy
BSP / Bromsulphthalein / sulfobromophthalein
B subtilis
BTL / bilateral tubal ligation
bucco- / *cheek*
buccal aspect / *toward cheek*
Budd-Chiari / *syndrome*
buddy taped / *injured finger immobilized by taping to next finger*
budesonide / *anti-inflammatory* / D
Buerger disease / thromboangiitis obliterans / *in thromboangiitis, pain of affected leg is often relieved by hanging it over the side of the bed*
buffy coat / *layer of white cells after centrifuging blood sample*
buflomedil / D
Buf-puf / *medicated cleanser for acne*
bulb ulceration
bulbocavernosus (Uro)
bulimic / bulimia nervosa / *constant and abnormal craving for food*
bullous (Derm) / *lesion*
Bumex / *diuretic* / D
BUN / blood-urea-nitrogen / *concentration of nitrogen in the form of urea (urine) found in the blood* / T

Additional Entries

---

bundle branch block (Cardio)
bundle of His (Cardio) / (syn.) atrioventricular bundle
Buprenex / *injectable* / *for pain* / D
Burkitt lymphoma / *usually, lesion in jaw or abdominal mass*
bursitis infrapatellar
burso- / *sac between bones that glide together*
burst of therapy / *prednisone*
BuSpar / *for anxiety disorders* / D
busulfan / *palliative for leukemia* / D
butalbital / Esgic / *sedative* / *for muscle contraction
    headache* / D
Butazolidin (discontinued 1992) / *antirheumatic* / D
Butisol / *sedative* / *hypnotic* / D
byssinosis (Pulm) / *type of obstructive airway disease* / *due
    to inhalation of textile dust*

B

Additional Entries

____

____

____

____

CA / cancer
CABG / coronary artery bypass graft
cac-, caci-, caco- / *bad* / *ill*
cachectic/-exia / *wasting away*
cacoethes / *a bad habit* / *a disorder*
CAD (Cardio) / coronary artery disease
cadaveric / *pertaining to a dead body*
Cafergot / *for migraine headaches* / D
caffeine / caffeinism
CAHC / chronic active hepatitis with cirrhosis
Caladryl / *lotion*
calamine lotion
Calan SR / verapamil hydrochloride / *slow channel blocker* / D
calc- / *heel* / *stone*
calcaneal area / *pertaining to heel*
calcaneus / *pertaining to heel*
calcar / *of lime*
Calciferol tablets (name changed to ergocalciferol) / vitamin D_2 /
    vitamin deficiency therapy
Calcijex / *for psoriasis* / D
Calcimar / *for post-menopausal osteoporosis* / D
calcinosis / *calcium deposits*
calcitonin / *calcium regulator* / D
calcium apatite stones / *type of mineral deposits*
calcium channel antagonists (Cardio) / D
calcium oxalate (Uro) / *kidney stone*
calculus / *pertaining to mineral deposits*
Caldwell-Luc operation / *incision to open maxillary sinus*
calicectasis / *dilatation of part of a kidney*
calix / *flower shaped* / *funnel shaped* / *part of kidney*
callosity / callus

C

Additional Entries

____

____

____

____

callus/-es / *thickening of skin*
   (Note: do not confuse with "callous" (adj.) / *emotionally hardened*)
Calm-X / *antiemetic* / D
Caltrate / *calcium supplement* / D
calvaria / *upper portion of skull / skullcap*
calvarium (incorrectly used for calvaria) / *see calvaria*
Calve-Perthes/-dis / *osteochondrosis of the femur*
calyceal/-es, caliceal/-es / *pertaining to the calix*
Cameron erosion (GI)
Camitz transfer
camptodactyly / *permanent flexion of fingers*
Campylobacter / *bacteria*
canalicular / *small, narrow, tubular channel*
canalization / *the formation of canals*
cancer / *any of several diseases in which cells grow abnormally*
Candida / *type of yeastlike fungus* / e.g., C. albicans
candidal pharyngitis
candidiasis (Gyn) / *yeast infection*
cannulation / *tube inserted into body cavity*
cantho- / *angle at end of eyelid*
cantharidin / *aphrodisiac ("Spanish fly")*
Cantil / *for peptic ulcer* / D
CAPD / continuous ambulatory peritoneal dialysis
Capitrol shampoo
Capener splint
capit-, cep- / *head* / e.g., de**capit**ate
capitellum / *head of humerus*
Capoten / captopril / *antihypertensive* / D
Capozide / captropril / *antihypertensive* / D
capsaicin (Zostrix) / *cream / for pain* / D [OTC]
capsid antigen

Additional Entries

____

____

____

____

capsules of Bowman (Uro)
capsulitis, adhesive / *limited movement in joint*
capsulotomy / *incision of a capsule, especially the eye*
captopril / Capoten (Cardio) / *antihypertensive* / D
caput, medusae / *varicose veins around the umbilicus*
Carafate / sucralfate / *for ulcer* / D
carbachol / isoptocarbachol (Oph) / *eye drops*
carbamazepine / Tegretol / *anticonvulsant* / *analgesic* / D
carbenicillin / *antibacterial* / D
Carbocaine / *local anesthetic* / D
carboplatin / Paraplatin / *antineoplastic* / D
carboxyhemoglobin
carcer- / *prison* / e.g., in**carcer**ate
carcin- (Onc) / *cancer* / e.g., **carcin**ogen
Cardene / nicardipine hydrochloride / *antihypertensive* / D
cardi-, cardio- (Cardio) / *heart* / e.g., **cardio**myopathy
cardiac cath / mid RCA / PDA / PL, D2
cardiobeeper
cardiogenic shock
cardiolipin / *antibody*
Cardiolite / *perfusion for cardiac imaging* / D
cardiomyopathy / *noninflammatory disease of the heart muscle*
Cardioquin / *antiarrhythmic* / D
cardioverter/-sion / *electric shock to restore normal heart rhythm*
Cardizem / *calcium channel blocker* / D
Cardura / *antihypertensive* / D
C2-3-4 area
Carey capsule
carina /-ae (pl.) / *ridgelike structure*
carious / *pertaining to caries* / *tooth decay*
carisoprodol / *skeletal muscle relaxant* / D

Additional Entries

____

____

____

____

Carmex ointment
carminative / *relieves flatulence*
Carmol HC / *moisturizer cream* / D
carnosity / *a fleshy growth*
caroticopharyngeal
carotid / *right and left common arteries that arise from the aorta*
carpal navicular / *in wrist* / *boat-shaped bone*
carpal tunnel syndrome
carpometacarpal / *bones of the hand and wrist*
carpopedal / *pertaining to both the wrist and the foot*
carposcaphoid
Carrington gel or pad
CARS (Pedi) / Children's Affective Rating Scale /
    also ... Childhood Autism Rating Scale
carteolol / *topical antiglaucoma agent* / D
cartilage / *fibrous connective tissue*
Cartrol / *beta blocker* / D
caruncula / *small, fleshy eminence* / *caruncle*
Castaderm / *topical antifungal* / D
CAT / computed axial tomography
cata-, **cath-** / *down* / *lower* / *under* / *complete* / e.g., **cath**eter
catabolism / *chemicals breaking down in the body*
Cataflam / diclofenac potassium / *nonsteroidal anti-inflammatory* / D
catalyst
catamenial / *pertaining to menses or to menstruation*
cataplexy / *abrupt muscular weakness triggered by happiness,*
    anger, fear or surprise
Catapres / *antihypertensive* / D
Catapres-TTS / *transdermal patch* / D
catarrh / *inflammation of mucous membrane*
catecholamines / *amines* / e.g., ephinephrine

Additional Entries

catheter / *tube that allows fluid to flow in or out of body /
    tube into urethra for urine drainage* / e.g., Hickman c.
catheterization
catholicon / *all inclusive*
cation / *(pronounced "cat-eye-on")*
cau- / *burn / sear* / e.g., **cau**terize
cauda- / *tail / tail-like appendage / lower (rear) end*
caudal lobe / *pertaining to the liver*
caudate / *having a tail*
cautery / *application of caustic or other agent to destroy
    living tissue*
cav- / *hollow*
Caverject / *for erectile dysfunction* / D
cavitary / *having a cavity*
cavum vergae
Cawthorne exercises / *for vertigo*
CBC / complete blood (cell) count
CC / chief complaint
C4-5 & C6
CCNU / chloroethylcyclohexylnitrosourea / *limustine* / D
CCPD / crystalline calcium pyrophosphate dihydrate / D
C-3/C.prime.3.normal
C. difficile toxin / Clostridium difficile / clostridial
C/D ratio / conjunctiva diagonalis (ratio)
cec- / *blind passage* / e.g., **cec**um
Ceclor / cefaclor / *antibiotic* / D
cecum / blind pouch / *cul-de-sac*
Cedax / *antibiotic for respiratory infections* / D
cefaclor / Ceclor / *antibiotic* / D
cefadroxil / Duricef / Ultracef / *antibiotic* / D
cefazolin / Ancef / Kefzol / Zolicef / *antibiotic* / D

C

Additional Entries

Cefobid / cefoperazone / *antibiotic* / D
cefotaxime / Claforan / *antibiotic* / D
cefpodoxime proxetil / Vantin / *antibiotic* / D
cefprozil / Cefzil / *antibiotic* / D
ceftazidime / URI / *antibiotic* / D
Ceftin / cefuroxime / *antibiotic* / D
ceftriaxone / Rocephin / *antibiotic* / for gonorrhea / D
cefuroxime / Ceftin /Axetil / *antibiotic* / D
CEI / continuous extravascular infusion
Celcet / D
-cele / *hernia* / *tumor or swelling* / e.g, hydro**cele**
Celestone 4 mg/ml/IM / *glucocorticoids*
celiac / *pertaining to the abdominal cavity*
celiac sprue / *intestinal malabsorption*
celio-, celo- / *abdomen* / *large cavity of the body*
celiotomy / abdominal section / laparotomy
cellulitis
Celsius / centigrade
centesis / *puncture* / e.g., amnio**centesis**
central enchondroma
centripetal / *moving toward a center*
centromere / *chromosome screen*
Centrum / *vitamin supplement*
Cepastat / *lozenges* / *mild local anesthetic*
cephal-, cephalo- / *head* / e.g., hydro**cephal**ic
cephalad / *toward head*
cephalexin / *antibiotic* / D
cephalization / *brain growth pattern*
cephalosporin / Ancef / *antibiotic* / D
cephradine / Velosef / *antibiotic* / D
cerebellar ataxia

Additional Entries

---

cerebr-, cerebi-, cerebro- / *brain* / e.g., **cerebr**al
cerebrovascular / *pertaining to blood supply to brain*
cerclage (Ortho) / *binding of certain fractures*
ceroma / *a waxy tumor*
ceruloplasmin / *lab*
cerumen / ceruminous / *earwax*
Cerumenex / *for dispersing earwax* / D
cervic- / *the neck* / *necklike structure*
cervical MRI / c. magnetic resonance imaging
cervical root syndrome
cervicitis (Gyn) / *inflammation of the cervix*
cervix / *constricted part of an organ*
cesarean / *lower uterine segment is incised*
cesium / *metallic element, atomic number 55*
cess / *go*
CGS units / centimeter-gram-second units
cGy / centi-gray
CH-(2.5.50)
Chagas disease / *from intestinal parasite*
chalazion (Oph)
chancre / *primary sore of syphilis*
Charcot-Marie-Tooth disease / *peroneal muscular atrophy*
Charcot changes (Pod) / *feet*
Chardack pacemaker
Charnley / *clamp*
Chediak-Higashi (Derm)
Cheetah / *ankle brace*
cheil- / *lip/s* / *of the face*
cheilectomy / *excision of a lip*
cheilitis/-osis
chein / *to pour*

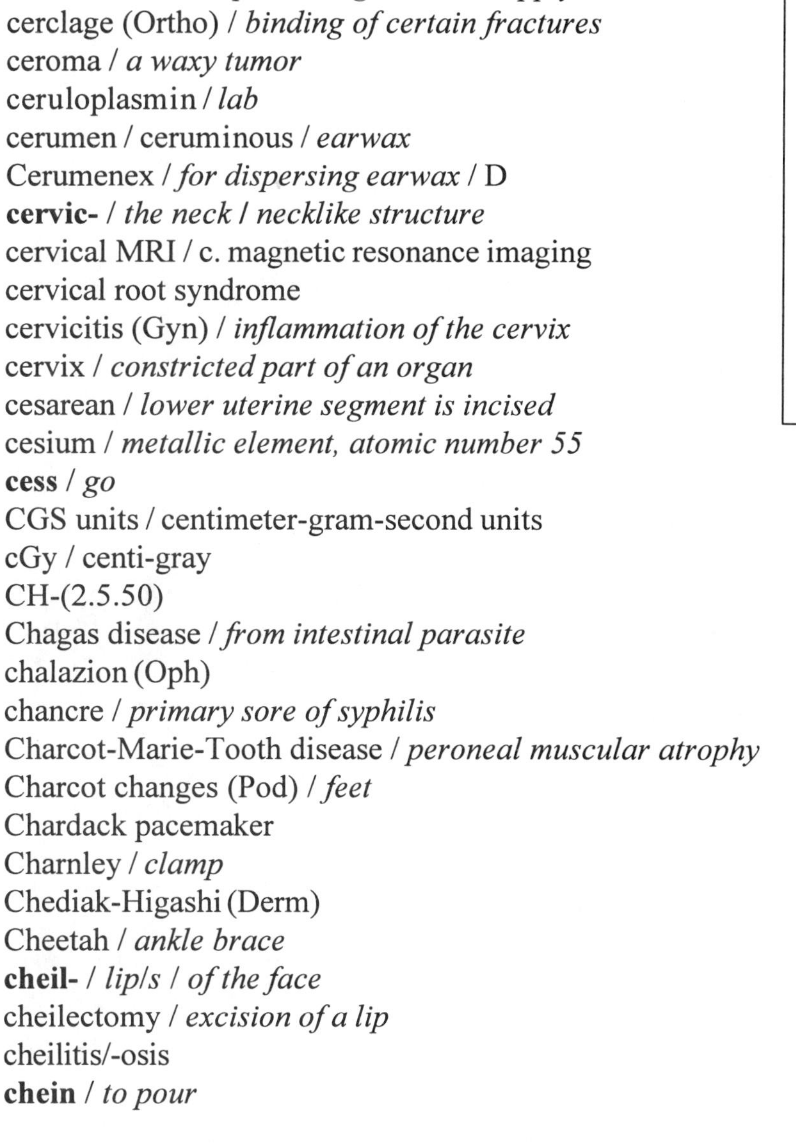

Additional Entries

cheir, chir / *the hand*
chelate/-ion / *complex chemical activity in the blood*
Chem-7
Chem-20 / Chemistry 20 profile
CHEMO:MVAC,TURBT.BCG
Chemzyme / *Chem-20*
Chenix / *for gallstones*
cherry angiomas / *tumors made up of blood vessels*
cherry-red spots / *In Tay-Sachs disease, a red spot in each retina*
chest thump / *sharp blow to precordial area of chest to restore
    normal heartbeat*
Cheyne-Stokes respirations
Chiari, osteotomy
Chiba / Jamshidi needle
Chilomastix / C. mesnili / chilomastigiasis
chir-, chiro- / *the hand*
chiropractic/-tor
Chlamydia pneumoniae / *bacteria that causes a mild pneumonia*
chloasma/-mata (Derm) / *melasma / blotchy brown macules, "mask
    of pregnancy" / also, at menopause and with birth control pills*
chloral hydrate / *hypnotic sedative* / D
chlorambucil / Leukeran / *antineoplastic* / D
chloramphenicol / *antibiotic* / D
Chloraseptic / *mild local anesthetic* / D
chlordiazepoxide / D
Chloromycetin (discontinued 1996) / *antibiotic* / D
chloroquine / *antimalarial* / *D*
chlorothiazide / *antihypertensive* / D
chlorpheniramine / *antihistamine* / D
chlorpromazine / Ormazine / Thorazine / *tranquilizer* / *antiemetic* /
    for relief of intractable hiccough / D

Additional Entries

____

____

____

____

chlorpropamide / *antidiabetic* / D
chlorthalidone / Hygroton / *antihypertensive* / D
Chlor-Trimeton / *antihistamine* / D
chlorzoxazone / *skeletal muscle relaxant* / D
Chlotrimazole...**NO!** (see Clotrimazole)
choanal / *funnel-shaped cavity*
cholangiocarcinoma / *malignancy of bile ducts*
cholangiogram / *radiographic record of bile ducts exam*
cholangiolytic
cholangiopancreatography
cholangitis / *inflammation of a bile duct*
chole- / *bile* / *gall*
cholecyst- / *bile sac* / *gallbladder*
cholecystectomy
cholecystitis
cholecystogram
choledochal / *pertaining to the common bile duct*
choledochoduodenostomy / jejunostomy
choledocholithiasis / *presence of gallstone in bile duct*
choledochostomy / *surgical opening and drainage of common bile duct*
Choledyl / *for cholelithiasis* / D
cholestasia/-is / *cessation of flow of bile*
cholesteatoma / *cystlike mass*
cholesterolemia / cholesteremia / *increased cholesterol in blood*
cholestyramine / *for hypercholesterolemia* / D
cholinergic urticaria / *rash, pertaining to nerve cells*
chondr- / *cartilage*
chondritis / *inflammation of cartilage*
chondrocalcinosis / *chronic arthritis similar to gout*
chondromalacia / *softness of cartilage, usually involving patella*

Additional Entries

____
____
____
____

CHOP / cyclophosphamide, hydroxydaunomycin, Oncovin
  (vincristine), and prednisone / *used in cancer therapy*
Chopart amputation / *disarticulation at the midtarsal joint*
chordee / *downward bowing of the penis*
chordoma / *rare tumor of vertebral column*
chorea / *irregular, involuntary movements*
chorea, Huntington / *inherited disease of central nervous system*
choreiform / *of the nature of chorea*
chorioretinitis (Oph) / *inflammation of choroid and retina*
choroidal nevus (Oph)
choroidopathy (Oph)
chromatin stain / *readily stainable part of cell nucleus*
chromium picolinate / *vitamin*
chronic / chronicity
chronotropic / *affecting the time or rate, as of the heart*
Chronulac / D
Churg-Strauss syndrome / *allergic granulomatous angiitis*
Chvostek and Trousseau sign / *facial muscles and nerve*
chyl / *gastric juice*
Chymex test / T
chymopapain (Ortho) / *enzyme* / *injection*
cicatricial pemphigus (Derm) / *skin disease*
cicatrix/-ization / *a scar*
cilia / *eyelash*
cilioretinal artery (Oph)
cilostazol (Vasc) / *drug study*
cimetidine / D
cimicosis (Derm) / *itching due to the bite of a bedbug*
cimino
CIN II
cine / *movement*

Additional Entries

____

____

____

____

cineangiocardiography / *motion picture of contrast medium passing through the heart*

cineangiography / *motion picture fluoroscopic images of blood vessels*

cineplasty / kineplasty / *plastic amputation where the stump is formed to be utilized for motor purposes*

cinnarrzine / *from Honduras* / D

Cinobac / *urinary antibacterial* / D

Cipro / ciprofloxacin / *antibiotic* / D

ciprofloxacin / D

circadian rhythm / *biological rhythms in a cycle of about 24 hours*

circum / *around* / *on all sides* / e.g., **circum**stantial

circumcised / *all or part of the foreskin removed*

circumduction / *circular movement of limb or of eye*

circumferential

circumoral paresthesias / *tingling of skin around mouth*

cirrhosis/-otic / *liver disease*

cirrus / (pl.) cirri / *slender, flexible appendage composed of fused cilia*

cirsomphalos / *varicose veins around the navel*

CIS / carcinoma in situ

cisapride / *peristaltic stimulant* / *for gastroesophageal reflux* / D

cisplatin / *anticancer* / D

Cis-Retinoic acid study

cisterna pontis / *cavity holding cerebrospinal fluid*

Citracal / *calcium supplement* / D

Citrobacter paracolon

Citrucel / *bulk laxative* / D

Civatte / poikiloderma of C.

CK Isoenzymes (CK-MB) (%MB)

Additional Entries

Claforan / *antibiotic for injection* / D
Clagett / *procedure*
clamidia...**NO!** (see "Chlamydia")
clarithromycin / Biaxin / *antibiotic* / D
Claritin / *nonsedating antihistamine* / *for chronic urticaria* / D
clas, **clad** / *break* / *destroy*
clasmatocyte / macrophage / *certain branched cells*
class III Pap
claudication (Cardio) / *limping* / *lameness*
clavicle (Ortho) / *collarbone*
clavulanate potassium / Augmentin / *amoxicillin* / D
clavus/-i (Pod) / *corn*
clawtoe deformities (Pod)
-cle / *small* / *little*
clean catch urine
Cleccin / *for acne* / *topical solution*
cleido / *collarbone*
cleidocranial / *clavicle and head*
cleidomastoid
clemastine fumarate / Tavist-D / *antihistamine* / D
Cleocin / clindamycin / *topical solution* / *for acne*
Cleocin T Gel / clindamycin / D
Climara / estradiol / *estrogen patch*
Clindex / *anxiolytic* / D
clinodactyly / *permanent deflection of one or more fingers*
Clinoril / sulindac / *nonsteroidal anti-inflammatory* / D
Clinoxide / Librax / *anxiolytic* / D
clitoral surgery (Gyn)
clival meningioma / *vascular tumor, cranial fossa*
cloaca / *the hindgut before division into rectum, bladder and genitals*
Clomid / clomiphene citrate / *ovulation stimulator* / D

Additional Entries

____
____
____
____

Clomid therapy / D
clomipramine / *antidepressant* / D
clonazepam / *anticonvulsant* / D
clonidine patch / *antihypertensive* / D
clonus, beats of / *muscle contraction*
clorazepate / *anxiolytic* / *mild tranquilizer* / D
closed reduction
Clostridium / *bacteria* / e.g., C. difficile; C. perfringens
Clotrimazole / *antifungal* / *vaginal* / D
cloxacillin / Cloxapen / Tegopen / *penicillin* / *antibacterial* / D
Clozaril (Psych) / *antipsychotic* / D
clubbing, cyanosis or edema / *physical exam of extremities,*
    "negative clubbing, cyanosis or edema"
clue cells / *epithelial cells* / in Gardnerella vaginitis
clus / *to close*
cm / centimeter
CMV titer / cytomegalovirus (titer)
CNS / central nervous system
C/O / complains of
coagulable
coagulase / *bacterial enzyme*
coalescence / *fusion or growing together of two or more body parts*
coal tar / *shampoo*
coapt/-ed / *to bring suture wound edges together*
CoA reductase / coenzyme A (reductase)
coarctation (Cardio) / *a condition of stricture on contraction*
Coban dressing
Coca-Cola
coccidioides / *fungi*
coccidiomycosis
-coccus / *bacterium*

Additional Entries

____

____

____

____

coccyalgia / *pain in coccyx*

coccyodynia / coccygodynia / coccygalgia / *pain in coccyx and neighboring region*

coccyx / *small bone at lower end of spine / tailbone*

cock-up / *wrist splint*

Codamine / *narcotic antitussive* / D

codeine / *antitussive / narcotic analgesic* / D

coel / *hollow* / e.g., coelom (pronounced "see-lum") / *cavity in an embryo between layers of mesoderm*

Cogan Reese syndrome (Oph)

Cogentin / *anticholinergic / antiparkinsonian* / D

Cognex / tacrine / *cognition adjuvant for Alzheimer disease* / D

cogwheel rigidity / *in Parkinson Disease*

coitus / *sexual intercourse*

Colabid / *for gout* / D

Colace / *stool softener* / D

ColBENEMID / *for gout* / D

colchicine / ColBENEMID / Proben-C / *for gout* / D

cold nodule

colectomy / *excision of a portion of the colon*

Colestid / *for lowering cholesterol* / D

colestipol / *lipid lowering drug*

coli / Escherichia (E. coli) / *bacteria*

colitis / *inflammation of the colon*

colla- / *glue / gelatinlike*

collagenolytic

collagenous colitis

Colles fracture (Ortho) / *wrist fracture, displaced*

colloid / *glutinous / resembling glue*

colloid goiter

colloid nodule

Additional Entries

____

____

____

____

colonoscopy
color flow Doppler
colovesical / *pertaining to colon and urinary bladder*
colpo- / *hollow* / *vagina*
colporrhaphy (Gyn) / *repair of vaginal rupture*
colposcopy (Gyn)
Coly-Mycin Otic (Oto) / *topical corticosteroidal anti-inflammatory antibiotic*
Combipres (Vasc) / *antihypertensive* / D
comedocarcinoma
comedo / (pl.) comedos or comedones / *primary lesion of acne* / *blackhead* / *zit*
Comhist LA / *decongestant* / *antihistamine* / D
commissurotomy / *incision to repair stenotic mitral valve*
Compazine / *antiemetic* / *tranquilizer* / D
compos mentis / *of sound mind* /
    and ... non compos mentis / *not of sound mind*
computed axial tomography / CAT scan / CT scan
concentric LVH / (concentric) left ventricular hypertrophy
concomitant esophageal spasm
concretion / *formation of solid material*
conductions / *transmission, as through nerves*
condyle / *a rounded projection on a bone*
Condylox / *for external genital warts* / D
condyloma/-mata acuminatum / *contagious growth on genitals*
coned-down view (Radiol)
confluent / *flowing together* / *blending into one*
conization / *excision of a cone of tissue*
conjunctivitis/-ival (Oph)
consensually / *eye reactions*
contra- / *against*

Additional Entries

____

____

____

____

contraindicated / *inappropriate treatment*
contractility / *capacity for becoming shorter*
contract for safety / *support system* / *for suicidal tendencies*
contrecoup / Fr. counterblow / *occurring on the opposite side* /
  damage at point opposite that at which blow was received /
  e.g., c. injury of the brain
Cooley anemia
cool mist humidifier
Coombs test / *antiglobulin* / T
Cooper ligament
COPD / chronic obstructive pulmonary disease
coprophilic / *pertaining to organisms that normally live in fecal*
  matter
coproporphyrin / *porphyrin in feces and urine*
cor / *heart* / e.g., c. triatriatum; c. bovinum; c. pulmonale
coracoacromial / *ligament*
coracoid / *shaped like a raven's beak*
coracoid process / *a process of the scapula*
cord, vocal
Cordarone / *antiarrhythmic* / D
cordis (L. *cor,* heart) / *pertaining to the heart* / e.g., diastasis c.
Cordis-Dow / *artificial kidney*
Cordran / *ointment* / *corticosteroid* / *antibiotic* / D
core antibody
core biloculare / *having two compartments*
Coreg / *for congestive heart failure (CHF)* / D
Co-Renite
Corgard / *antihypertensive* / *antianginal* / D
Coricidin D / *decongestant* / *antihistamine* / D
Cormax / *for scalp itch* / D
corne- / *horny* / *hornlike*

Additional Entries

---

corneae arcus (Oph)
corona radiata (Neuro) / *a fiber mass in the cerebral cortex*
corporis, tinea (Derm) / *ringworm of body*
cor pulmonale / (pl.) cor pulmonalia / *hypertrophy or failure of right ventricle from lung or pulmonary vessel disorder*
corpus / corporis / (pl.) corpora / *a body or mass* / *main part of an organ* / e.g., c. albicans; c. corpora; c. callosum
corpuscular / *pertaining to a small mass, body or blood cell*
corpus hemorrhagicum / *ovarian follicle containing blood*
correctable/-ible
Correctol (discontinued 1996) / *laxative*
Cortef / *glucocorticoids* / D
cortical / *pertaining to a cortex*
cortical shots
corticosteroid
Cortifoam / *for ulcerative proctitis* / D
cortisol / *hydrocortisone* / D
cortisone / *glucocorticoid* / D
Cortisporin Otic Solution (ENT) / *ear drops* / *corticosteroidal anti-inflammatory* / D
Cortrosyn / injection / *for multiple sclerosis* / *for infantile spasms* / D
coruscation (Oph) / *flashes of light*
Coryne bacterium
coryza / *catarrh of nasal membrane with profuse discharge*
Corzide / *antihypertensive* / D
cost- / *rib* / *costal* / *chondrocostal*
costal / *ribs*
Costen syndrome / *temporomandibular dysfunction*
costo- / *the ribs*
costochondral/-itis
costophrenic angle

Additional Entries

____
____
____
____

costovertebral angle
cosyntropin / *adrenocorticotropic hormone*
Cotrel traction / *instrumentation* / *rod*
cotyledon (Gyn) / *placental unit* / e.g., fetal c.; maternal c.
Coulter / *lab*
Coumadin / *anticoagulant* / D
coup de sabre / *scalp scleroderma that causes scarring*
couplets
Cournand cardiac catheter
Covera HS/240 mg / *antihypertensive* / *antianginal* / D
Coversil
coxa magna / femur magna
coxa valga / *hip deformity*
coxa vara luxans
coxodynia / coxalgia / *pain in the hip joint*
coxsackievirus / Coxsackie virus (from Coxsackie, N.Y.) / *virus
    producing disease resembling polio, but without paralysis*
Cozaar / *antihypertensive* / *angiotensin blocker* / D
CPAP / continuous positive airway pressure / *for sleep apnea*
C-peptide levels / *lab*
CPK / creatine phosphokinase / *elevated in muscular dystrophy* / T
CPR / cardiopulmonary resuscitation
crani- / *skull*
cranial nerves, II-XII / *(there are 12 paired cranial nerves)*
craniopharyngioma
craniocaudad
C-reactive protein / *a globulin*
creatinine PAH clearance / para-aminohippurate
creatinine phosphokinase
cremaster/-ic muscle(s) / *muscles that retract the testicles*
Creon / *digestive enzymes* / D

Additional Entries

____

____

____

____

crepitant/-ation / *rattling* / *cracking*

crepitus/-ation / *crackling sound in tissue* / *grating of broken bones*

crescendo/decrescendo, ejection murmur (Cardio)

cret / *grow*

CREST syndrome / *scleroderma*

CRF / corticotropin-releasing factor

CRST / cyanosis, redness, scleroderma, telangiectasis / *in Raynaud phenomenon* / *response to cold*

cricoarytenoid/-eous / *pertaining to throat cartilages*

cricoid cartilage

cricopharyngeal

cricopharyngeous, ring

-crine / *to secrete*

Crohn disease (GI) / *involving terminal ileum*

cromolyn / *inhaler* / *prophylactic antiasthmatic*

CRP / C-reactive protein

CRPA / C-reactive protein antiserum

cruciate, anterior / *ligaments*

cruciferous / *vegetables of the mustard family* / e.g., brussels sprouts, broccoli, cabbage, turnips

crural / *the leg, thigh, or any anatomical structure resembling a leg*

cryo-, cry-, crymo- / *cold* / e.g., **cryo**gen

Cryocrit

cryocautery / *for removal of skin keratoses*

cryofibrinogen (Hemo) / *abnormal type fibrinogen rarely found in blood*

cryofibrinogenemia (Hemo) / *cryofibrinogen in blood*

cryoglobulinemia (Hemo)/*abnormal levels of cryoglobulin in blood*

cryothalamectomy / *destruction of thalamus by applying extreme cold*

Additional Entries

____

____

____

____

cryoretinopexy
crypt-, crypto-, cry-, / *hidden* / *obscure* / *without apparent cause*
cryptococcal meningitis
cryptorchidism / *failure of testis or testes to descend into scrotum*
cryptosis
C&S / culture and sensitivity / T
CSF / cerebrospinal fluid
CT / computed tomography
CT of abdomen / computed tomography (of abdomen)
ctenoids / (pronounced "ten-oids")
C-Terminal
CTS / carpal tunnel syndrome / e.g., bilateral c. t. s.
cubital fossa (Ortho)
cubitus (Ortho) / *elbow*
cuff / *aneroid blood pressure cuff*
cuff, rotator (Ortho) / *of shoulder*
cul-de-sac / *a pouch* / *tubular cavity closed at one end*
culdocentesis / *aspiration of fluid from cul-de-sac*
cuneiform / *wedge-shaped*
cup-to-disc ratio (Oph)
Curasol / *salve*
Curretab / *for abnormal uterine bleeding* / D
curet / *spoon-shaped instrument*
curettage / D&C / dilatation and curettage
curettement / *the removal of material from the wall of a cavity*
curvilinear incision
Cushing syndrome / *disorder resulting from abnormal levels of*
  cortisol
  also ... Cushing medicamentosus / *symptoms of C. syndrome,*
  such as peptic ulcer, caused by chronic administration of large
  doses of any steroid

Additional Entries

____

____

____

____

cushingoid
cut- / *skin*
cutis marmorata (Derm) / *skin mottling from cold*
Cutivate / *topical corticosteroidal anti-inflammatory* / D
CVA / cardiovascular accident
   also ... cerebrovascular accident
cyan- / *dark blue* / e.g., **cyan**osis
cyclandelate / Cyclospasmol / *peripheral vasodilator* / D
cycling dialysis
cyclobenzaprine / Flexeril / *muscle relaxant* / D
Cyclogyl / cyclopentolate hydrochloride / *eye drops* / D
cyclophosphamide / *antineoplastic* / *immunosuppressive* / D
cyclosporin / *immunosuppressive* / D
cyclothymia/-ic / *mental disorder characterized by extreme mood swings*
Cycrin / *for abnormal uterine bleeding* / D
Cylert / pemoline / *stimulant for attention deficit hyperactive disorders* / D
cyst- / *sac* / *bladder*
cyst, inclusion / epidermal cyst
cysticercosis / *worm*
cystitis / *inflammation of the bladder*
cystine / *sulfur-containing amino acid*
cystinemia / *presence of cystine in blood*
cystinosis / *inherited disease characterized by abnormal deposits of cystine in body tissues*
cystinuria / *presence of cystine in urine*
cystocele / *hernia of the bladder, usually into vagina and introitus*
cystocytoma / *a fibroma*
cystoid macular edema (Oph)

Additional Entries

---

cystometrics (Uro)
cystosarcoma phylloides
cystoscopy (Uro)
Cystospaz / *anticholinergic* / *antispasmodic* / D
cystourethrogram (Uro)
cyto-, cyt- / *a cell*
cytobrush (Gyn) / *used for Pap*
cytogenetics / *study of cell formation, structure and function*
cytoid / *resembling a cell*
cytomegalovirus / CMV
Cytomel / misoprostol / *thyroid hormone* / D
cytometric (Chemo) / *flow studies*
Cytosar-U / *antineoplastic for leukemias* / D
cytosine arabinoside / *antiviral* / *antineoplastic* / D
Cytotec / misoprostol / *for prevention of NSAID-induced gastric
    ulcers* / D

Additional Entries

D5 / *normal saline* / *D5 and half = D5 and 0.5 NS*
dacro-, dacry- / *tears* / *lacrimal sac or duct*
dactyl / *finger* / *toe*
Dalmane / flurazepam HCL / *sedative* / *hypnotic* / D
danazol / Danocrine / *anterior pituitary suppressant* / D
Dandy-Walker syndrome / *in hydrocephalus*
Danocrine / danazol / *androgen for endometriosis* / D
dapsone / Avlosulfon / *bactericidal* / D
Darco shoe
Darier disease (Derm)
Darvocet-N 100 / *narcotic analgesic* / D
Darvon / propoxyphene / *narcotic analgesic* / D
daunomycin / *antibiotic antineoplastic* / D
daunorubicin / *antibiotic antineoplastic* / D
Davol PermCath
Daypro / oxaprozin / *for arthritis* / *NSAID, nonsteroidal anti-inflammatory drug* / D
DayQuil / *antitussic* / *decongestant* / D [OTC]
D&C / dilatation and curettage
DC / discontinue
DDAVP / *trademark for preparation of desmopressin* / D
DDT / dichlorodiphenyltrichloroethane
debridement / *removal of dead tissue or foreign matter from wound*
Debrox (ENT) / *drops for earwax dispersion*
debulking / *removal of most of a lesion*
Decadron / dexamethasone / *glucocorticoids* / D
Deca-Durabolin injection / nandrolone / *steroid for anemia of renal insufficiency* / D
2-D echo (Cardio) / T
Declomycin / demeclocycline / *broad-spectrum antibiotic* / D
Deconamine / *decongestant* / *antihistamine* / D

D

Additional Entries

____

____

____

____

decreased pinprick / *a decrease in sensation*
decrement / *decrease*
decubitus/-iti / *pressure sores*
deep tendon reflexes
defervescent / *reduce fever*
degenerative joint disease / DJD
deglutition / *the act of swallowing*
dehisce/-ence / *gape / wound splitting open*
Delestrogen / ERT / *estrogen replacement therapy* / D
Delsym / *cough medicine*
Deltasone / *vaginal / corticosteroid / prednisone* / D
Demadex / torsemide / *loop diuretic* / D
demarcation / *setting limits or boundaries*
demeclocycline / *antibacterial* / D
dementia / *loss of cognitive and intellectual functions*
Demerol / *narcotic analgesic* / D
demise / *death*
Demulen 1/35 / *birth control pill*
demyelination/-ization / *loss of myelin within central nervous system*
dendr- / *tree / treelike / branching*
dendrite (CNS) / *one of the two types of branching protoplasmic
   processes of nerve cells (the other is the axon)* / e.g., apical d.
dengue fever
dense cataracts (Oph)
dent- / *teeth*
dentition / *natural teeth*
denudation / *laying bare*
Depakote / *anticonvulsant / antipsychotic / migraine preventative* / D
Depakene / *antiepileptic / anticonvulsant* / D
dependent / *the leg is hanging down*
   also ... d. rubor / *redness of lower legs from hanging down*

Additional Entries

____
____
____
____

depigmentation / *removal of pigment, especially from skin, by chemical or physical means*

depigmented rash of tinea versicolor (Derm)

Depo-Estradiol / *hormone replacement* / *for post-meno-pausal disorders* / D

Depo-Medrol 40 mg/ml

Depo-Provera / *long-term injectable contraceptive* / D

Depo-Testosterone / *androgen replacement* / *for breast cancer* / D

Deponit Patch / nitroglycerin / *antianginal* / D

deprenyl / selegiline / *antiparkinsonian* / D

deQuervain disease / *tenosynovitis* / *of thumb*

derm-, derma- / *the skin*

dermal lymphocytic (Derm)

dermal nevi (Derm)

dermatitis, escharotic (Derm)

dermatofibroma (Derm) / *slow growing, benign skin nodule*

dermatographism (Derm)/ *a form of urticaria with whealing*

dermatologic

dermatome/-tomal / *an instrument for cutting thin skin slices for skin grafts*

dermatomycosis (Derm) / *fungus infection*

dermatomyositis (Derm) / *progressive condition characterized by muscle weakness and skin rash*

dermoid / (syn.) dermoid cyst / *resembling skin*

derotative righting (Ortho)/ *reflex*

DES / diethylstilbestrol / stilbestrol / *estrogen* / *for inoperable breast and prostate cancer* / D

descensus / *falling* / *descending* / e.g., d. testis; d. uteri

Desenex / *topical antifungal* / D

desensitization

Additional Entries

---

desferrioxamine / mesylate / *antidote to iron poisoning* / *iron chelating agent* / D
desiccated thyroid / *treatment of a tumor by drying it up* / D
desipramine / *antidepressant* / D
-desis / *binding* / *fusion* / *surgical union* / e.g., arthro**desis** / *of a joint*
Desitin / *ointment* / *emollient* / *astringent* / *antiseptic*
desmoid tumor / *fibromatous tumor of abdominal wall*
desmopressin acetate / DDAVP / *nasal spray* / *pituitary antidiuretic hormone* / D
Desogen / *oral contraceptive* / D
Desonide / *lotion* / *corticosteroid anti-inflammatory* / D
DesOwen / desonide / *topical corticosteroid anti-inflammatory* / D
Desoxyn / methamphetamine / *central nervous system stimulant* / D
desquamation/-ating / *to shed* / *peel* / *scale off*
Desquam / benzoyl peroxide / *for acne* / D
Desyrel / trazodone / *antidepressant* / D
detrusor / *muscle that can expel a substance*
dexamethasone / *corticosteroid* / D
dexa scan
Dexedrine / *amphetamine* / *CNS stimulant* / *for attention deficit disorder* (ADD) / D
dextromethorphan / *antitussive* / D
dextroscoliotic
DH / delayed hypersensitivity
DHEA / dihydroepiandrosterone / *sulfate test* / T
dia- / *through* / *throughout* / *completely*
DiaBeta / glyburide / *sulfonylurea antidiabetic* / D
diabetes insipidus
diabetes mellitus
Diabinese / chlorpropamide / *antidiabetic* / D

Additional Entries

____

____

____

____

diabrosis / *eating through* / *a corrosion causing perforation of a vessel or organ*

diabrotic / *corrosive*

diadochokinesia/-is (Ortho) / *normal limb movement*

diafram...**NO!** (see "diaphragm")

dialyze/-s / *to perform dialysis*

diastasis cordis (Cardio) / *any period of mechanical inactivity of the heart*

Diamond-Blackfan syndrome (Hemo)

Diamox / acetazolamide / *anticonvulsant* / D

Dianeal (discontinued 1996) / *peritoneal dialysis solution* / D

diaphoresis / *perspiration*

diaphragm / *partition between abdomen and thoracic cavities*

diaphragmatic hernia

diaphram...**NO!** (see "diaphragm")

diapiresis / *minute particles of suspended matter passing through unruptured walls of blood vessels*

diarrhea / diarrheal

diastasis recti / *separation of abdominal muscles from midline*

diastematomyelia / *pertaining to division of spinal cord*

diastolic (Cardio) / *bottom blood pressure number*

diathesis / *disposed to develop diseases or structural anomalies*

diazepam / Dizac injection / Valium / *anxiolytic* / D

diclofenac potassium / *antiarthritic*

dicloxacillin / Penicillin / *antibacterial* / D

dicyclomine / *anticholinergic* / D

Didronel / etidronate disodium / *bone resorption suppressant* / D

dienestrol / dienoestrol / *estrogen* / *vaginal cream* / D

diethylstilbestrol / DES / Stilphostrol / *estrogen* / *for inoperative breast and prostate cancer* / D

Additional Entries

____

____

____

____

dietitian
Dieulofois lesion
difficile
diffuse lumbosacral tenderness (Ortho)
Diflucan / *systemic antifungal* / D
digit / *finger* / *toe*
digoxin / Lanoxicaps / Lanoxin / *cardiac glycoside* / D
dihydroergotamine mesylate / D.H.E. 45 injection / *for rapid control of migraines* / D
dihydropteridine
diiodohydroxyquinoline / *amebicide* / *antimicrobial* / D
Dilacor / diltiazem / *antihypertensive* / *antianginal* / D
Dilantin / phenytoin / *anticonvulsant* / D
dilatation and curettage / D&C
Dilatrate-SR / isosorbide dinitrate / *antianginal* / D
Dilaudid / hydromorphone / *narcotic analgesic* / D
diltiazem / Cardizem / *coronary vasodilator* / *calcium channel blocker* / D
Dimetane / *antihistamine* / D
Dimetapp / *decongestant* / *antihistamine* / D
diminution / *diminishing*
Dipentum / olsalazine / *anti-inflammatory for ulcerative colitis* / D
diphenhydramine / *antihistamine* / *motion sickness relief* / D
diphtheroids
DIP joint / distal interphalangeal joint / *joint nearest end of fingers and toes*
diplegia / *double hemiplegia*
diplococcus/-i (pl.) / *bacteria*
diplopia / *double vision*
Diprivan / *general anesthetic emulsion for IV* / D
Diprolene / *topical corticosteroid* / D

Additional Entries

Diprosone / *topical corticosteroid* / D
dips- / *thirst*
dipyridamole / *coronary vasodilator* / *antiplatelet agent* / D
Dipy-thal / dipyridamole thallium / *for scan*
dis- / *in two* / *apart* / *asunder* / *opposite of*
Disalcid / *analgesic* / D
disarticulation (Ortho) / *amputation of limb through a joint, without cutting bone*
discogenic (Ortho)
discoid lupus
disequilibrium
DISIDA scan / diisopropyliminodiacetic acid / *for scan*
diskectomy (Ortho)
diskitis (Ortho)
disomic disorder
dist- / *far*
distal interphalangeal joint (Ortho) / *toes*
distal to proximal / *farthest to nearest*
distention/-sion / *distended* / *stretched*
Ditropan / oxybutynin / *urinary antispasmodic for neurogenic bladder* / D
Diulo (discontinued 1993) / *diuretic* / D
diuresed (Uro)
diuresis (Uro) / *excretion of urine*
diuretic (Uro) / *an agent that increases urination*
Diuril / *diuretic* / D
diverticulosis coli
diverticulum/-ula / *pouch or sac opening from an organ*
Dix-Hallpike / T
dizziness simulation battery / T
DJD / degenerative joint disease

D

Additional Entries

____

____

____

____

DLCO / PFT / diffusing capacity (of) lung (for) carbon monoxide / T
D5NS-DF / *normal saline*
DOB / date of birth
dobutamine / *cardiotonic / vasopressor for shock* / D
dobutamine spiff / *three-day hospital treatment to "spiff" up the heart*
Dobutrex / dobutamine / *IV vasopressor for cardiac shock*
docusate / *stool softener* / D
Dolobid / diflunisal / *analgesic / antiarthritic / anti-inflammatory* /D
domperidone study / *antiemetic*
dominant / *right hand*
Domeboro soaks / *for tinea*
Donnagel / *antidiarrheal* / D
Donnatal Extentabs / *anticholinergic / sedative* / D
Doppler / *ultrasonography /*
    also ... color flow Doppler imaging
Doral / *sedative / hypnotic* / D
Dorcol / *pediatric nasal decongestant* / D
dors- / *the back side / posterior*
dorsal column stimulator
dorsalgia / rachialgia / *pain in the back*
dorsal-recumbent / *lying on one's back*
dorsalis / *position closer to the back surface*
dorsiflexors / *flexion toward the extensor aspect*
dorsum / *back of / posterior*
Doryx / doxycycline / *tetracycline-type antibiotic* / D
Dostinex / *for hyperprolactinemia* / D
douloureux, tic / *trigeminal neuralgia*
Dovonex (Derm) / *topical antipsoriatic* / D
Down syndrome / mongolism
doxepin / *antidepressant* / D

Additional Entries

____

____

____

____

Doxidan / docusate / phenolphthalein / *stool softener* / *for constipation* / D

doxorubicin / *antibiotic antineoplastic* / D

doxycycline / *bacteriostatic* / *antirickettsial* / D

DPT / diphtheria, pertussis and tetanus

Dr. Akin's / *mouthwash*

Dramamine / *antinauseant* / *motion sickness preventative* / D

drawer sign (Ortho) / *knees*

DRG / diagnosis related group

Drisdol / *vitamin deficiency therapy* / D

Drixoral / *decongestant* / *antihistamine* / D

drift / pronator / *pertaining to muscles*

Dr. Scholl / *foot products*

dronabinol / THC / thc / *antinauseal* / D

drusen (Oph) / *plaque*

Drysol / *astringent for hyperhidrosis* / D

dry weight

dT / *immunizations* / *diphtheria tetanus toxoids (see Td)*

DTIC-Dome / dacarbazine / *antineoplastic* / *for metastatic malignant melanoma* / D

DTR / deep tendon reflexes

DuoDerm dressing / *occlusive wound dressing*

DUB / dysfunctional uterine bleeding

Dubowitz / *pediatric scale*

Duchenne / *muscular dystrophy*

duct / *tube* / *channel*

Dukes C / *stage of colon cancer*

dumping syndrome / postgastrectomy s. (GI) / *sweating and weakness after eating* / *caused by rapid passage (dumping) of large amounts of food into small intestine*

Dulcolax / *stimulant laxative* / D

Additional Entries

---

duodenum/-al / *part of small intestine from stomach to jejunum*
duodenitis / *inflammation of duodenum*
Duoderm / *adhesive bandages* / D
DuoFilm / *topical keratolytic* / D
DuoPlant / *topical keratolytic* / *for plantar warts* / D
Dupuytren contractures / *flexion deformity of a finger*
dura- / *hard*
Duratuss / *decongestant* / *expectorant* / D
Dura-Vent / *decongestant* / *antihistamine* / D
Duricef / *cephalosporin-type antibiotic* / D
Durkan sign / *carpal tunnel* / T
dx / *diagnosis*
Dyazide / *diuretic* / *antihypertensive* / D
Dymelor / *for diabetes* / D
dyn-, odyn-, odyno- / *pain* / e.g., **odyno**phagia
DynaCirc / isradipine / *antihypertensive* / D
dynam- / *power* / *force* / *energy* / e.g., **dynam**ic
Dynapen / *bacterial antibiotic* / D
dynophagia...**NO!** (see "odynophagia")
Dyrenium / *potassium-sparing diuretic* / D
dys- / *bad* / *out of order* / *difficult* / *opposite*
dysarthria/-ic / *disturbance of speech and language*
dyscrasia / *morbid feelings* / *due to abnormal blood substances*
dysdiadochokinesia/-esis / *from impairment, inability to perform
    rapidly alternating movements*
dysesthesia / *loss or lack of sensation*
dysfunction
dyshidrosis/-es / *vesicular eruption on hands and feet* (from
    hidrosis / *sweating)*
dyskinesia / *difficulty doing voluntary movements*
dyslipidemia

Additional Entries

____

____

____

____

dysmenorrhea / *painful menstruation*
dysmetria / *difficulty controlling movements*
dysmorphic / *abnormal shape*
dysmotility / *difficulty controlling spontaneous movement*
dyspareunia / *painful coitus*
dyspepsia / *upset stomach / pain in stomach*
dysphagia / *difficulty swallowing*
dysphasia / *difficulty speaking*
dysphoria / *disquiet-malaise*
dysplasia / *abnormal cell growth*
dysplastic / *pertaining to dysplasia*
dyspnea/-ic / *difficult breathing*
dysraphism / *tube closure / defective fusion of neural tube*
dysrhythmia / *abnormal rhythm*
dysthymia / *depression*
dysthymic disorder / *chronic depressed mood*
dystonia/-ic / *abnormal tonicity of tissues*
dystrophy/-ic / *"bad nourishment" / changes that may result from defective nutrition of a tissue or organ*
dysuria / *difficult urination / painful urination*
D-xylose / *test for fat malabsorption / T*

D

Additional Entries

____

____

____

____

ear loop / *used for cerumen impaction*
early missed AB / *an explanation for positive home pregnancy test, followed by negative lab pregnancy test*
Eaton-Lambert syndrome / *myesthenialike condition in which the weakness affects the limbs*
Ebstein's anomaly (Cardio) / *atrial septal defect*
EBV / Epstein-Barr virus
ecchymosis / *purple skin discoloration caused by blood passing from a vessel into the skin*
ECG / EKG / electrocardiogram
echocardiogram (Cardio)
echogenic/-ity
echolalia / *involuntary repetition of a word or phrase spoken by another*
eclampsia / *convulsion(s) in a pregnant woman with pre-eclampsia*
E. coli / Escherichia coli / *bacterium*
econazole nitrate / Spectazole / *antifungal* / D
ectasia / *dilatation*
-ectasia, -ectasis / *expansion* / *stretching out* / *enlargement* / *dilatation*
ectatic / *pertaining to ectasis*
ecto- / *outside*
-ectomy / *removal of all or part of*
ectopia/-ic / *organ or body part that is out of place*
ectro- / *congenital absence of a part*
ectrocheiry / ectrochiry / *absence of part or all of a hand*
ectropion (Oph)
Ecuador
eczema craquelé (Derm)
eczema, nummular (Derm)
eczematoid (Derm)

Additional Entries

____

____

____

____

ED / effective dose
Edecrin / *loop diuretic* / D
edema / *excessive fluid* / *pitting*
edematous
edentulous / *toothless*
E.E.S. 400 Filmtab / *macrolide antibiotic* / D
efferent / *fluid or nerve impulse flowing **outward***
    (opposite) afferent / fluid or nerve impulse flowing ***inward***
Effexor / *antidepressant* / D
effusion / *fluid escape into a body part or tissue*
Efudex / fluorouracil / *cream* / *antimetabolic antineoplastic* / *for*
    actinic keratoses and basal cell carcinomas / D
EGD / Esophago Gastro Duodenoscopy
egophony / egobronchophony
Ehlers-Danlos syndrome / *inherited disorders of the connective*
    tissue
ejection fraction of the heart (Cardio)
EKG / ECG / electrocardiogram
Elastoplast wrap
Elavil / *tricyclic antidepressant* / D
Eldepryl / *antiparkinsonian* / D
electrocardiogram (12-lead) (Cardio)
electrodesiccated
electrogalvanic
electrolyte / *any compound that, in solution, conducts electricity*
electromyogram
electrophoresis / capillary zone
Elimite / cream / *for scabies* / D
ELISA / enzyme-linked immunoadsorbent assay / *test for H. pylori* / T
ellipse / *spherical shape*
Ellipse compact spacer

Additional Entries

____

____

____

____

elliptocyte / *oval-shaped red cells*
Elocon / *topical corticosteroid* / D
Elspar / *adjunct for acute lymphocytic leukemia* / D
EMB / eosin methylene blue
embolization
embolus/-ic / *clotted blood or other formed elements that plug a blood vessel*
-emesis / *vomiting*
Emetrol / *antinauseant* / *antiemetic* / D
EMG / electromyogram
emphysema (Pulm)
empiric / *rational* / *based on testing*
empyema / *pus in a body cavity*
E-Mycin / *macrolide antibiotic* / D
enalapril maleate / Vaseretic / *for hypertension* / D
enameloblastoma / *tumor of enamel buds or germ cells* / *tumor of the jaw formed from remnants of tooth enamel germ cells*
encainide HCl / Enkaid / *antiarrhythmic* / D
enchondroma / *benign growth of cartilage arising in a bone*
encopresis / *incontinence of feces not due to organic defect or illness*
end-, endo- / *inside* / *within inner lining* / *absorbing* / *containing*
Endal / *decongestant* / *expectorant* / D
endarterectomy / *excision of diseased matter from an artery, often in a carotid artery*
end expiratory wheezes
endocarditis (Cardio) / *inflammation of the endocardium*
endocrine system / *glands that secrete hormones and enzymes*
endogenous depression / *arising from within*
Endolimax / *small nonpathogenic intestinal parasitic amebae*
endometrial (Gyn) / *pertaining to the lining of the uterus*

E

Additional Entries

endometriosis (Gyn) / *ectopic growth of endometrial tissue*
endometrioma (Gyn) / *mass of tissue*
endoperimyocarditis (Cardio)
end organs
endoscope/-y / *instrument for examinations*
endplate
end respiratory crackles
end terminal PTH / (end terminal) parathyroid hormone
Enduron / *diuretic / antihypertensive* / D
Enkaid / encainide / D
en plaques / *in the form of a plaque or plate*
Ensure / *dietary supplement*
ENT / ears, nose (and) throat
Entamoeba coli / *ameboid protozoa parasite*
enter-, entero- / *intestines*
Enterobacter / *bacteria*
enterocele (Gyn) / *hernial protrusion*
Enterococcus faecalis
enterogastritis / gastroenteritis (GI) / *inflammation of mucous membranes of stomach and intestine*
enterohepatic / *pertaining to the intestines and the liver*
Entex LA / Entex PSE / *decongestant / expectorant* / D
enthesis / *use of synthetic or other material to replace lost tissue*
enthesopathy / *disease process at point of insertion of muscle tendons into bones*
enucleated/-tion / *to remove entirely*
enuresis / *bedwetting*
EOM (ENT) / external otitis media
EOMI HEENT (Oph) / extraocular muscles intact in HEENT exam (HEENT: head, eyes, ears, nose and throat)
eosinophil / eosinophilic leukocyte

Additional Entries

---

eosinophilia / *large number of eosinophils in the blood, readily stained with eosin*

eparterial / *located over or above an artery*

ependymoma (Neuro) / *a glioma*

ephedrine / adrenaline / *bronchodilator / vasopressor for shock* / D

ephelis / (pl.) ephelides / freckle

epi- / *upon / over/ outer covering* / e.g., **epi**dermis

EPI / exocrine pancreatic insufficiency

epiandrosterone / *androgenic hormone normally in urine*

epicondyle (Ortho) / *projection from a long bone*

epicondylitis (Ortho)

epicondylotomy (Ortho)

epicrisis / *secondary crisis following the initial critical stage of a disease*

epidermoid (Onc) / *resembling epidermis / a tumor growing from abnormal epidermal cells* / e.g., e. carcinoma

epididymal/-is/-itis / *pertaining to the testes*

Epifoam / *topical corticosteroid / aerosol foam local anesthetic* / D

epigastrium / epigastric region

epiglottis (ENT) / *elastic cartilage at the root of the tongue*

epileptic/-sy (Neuro) / *chronic brain dysfunction, often associated with altered consciousness*

Epilyt Cream / *moisturizer / emollient* / D

epinephrine 1:1000

epinephrine / Sus-phrine / *adrenaline / vasoconstrictor / bronchodilator* / D

EpiPen / *used in emergency treatment of anaphylaxis* / D

epiphysial / epiphyseal (Ortho)

epiphysiodesis (Ortho)

epiphysis (Ortho) / *part of a long bone*

Additional Entries

epiploic / omental/-um (GI) / *pertaining to a fold of peritoneum passing from the stomach to another abdominal organ*

epiretinal (Oph)

epis / *epithelial cells*

episcleritis / *inflammation of episcleral connective tissue*

episiotomy (Gyn) / *surgical incision into perineum and vagina to prevent tearing during delivery*

episode, lone / *only happened once*

epistasis / *suppression of any discharge*

epistaxis / *nosebleed*

epithelial (Derm)

Epitol / *pain control for postherpetic neuralgia* / D

epitrochlear / *the inner condyle of the humerus*

Epogen / opoetin alfa / *in dialysis* / *stimulates red blood cell production for anemia of end-stage renal disase*

eponychial/-ium / *part of a toenail*

eponym / *a disease, instrument, operation or procedure, or other object named after the person who first discovered or described it*

EPR / electron paramagnetic resonance

Epstein-Barr / *a virus*

epulis / *a fibrous sarcomatous tumor of the lower jaw*

Equagesic / *analgesic* / *antipyretic* / *anxiolytic* / D

equinus deformity / *"like a horse"* / e.g., talipes equinus / *permanent extension of foot, only ball rests on the ground*

ERCP / endoscopic retrograde cholangiopancreatography

Ercaf / ergotamine derivatives / *for headaches* / D

erector spinae (Ortho)

Erecaid / D

erethism / *abnormal state of excitement or irritation*

Erex / D

Additional Entries

---

ergocalciferol (formerly Calciferol) / *vitamin deficiency therapy / vitamin D$_2$*

ergoloid mesylates / *cognition for age-related mental decline* / D

ergometer / dynamometer / *device for measuring muscular power*

ergonovine / *chemical*

Ergostat (discontinued 1996) / *sublingual / migraine-specific vasoconstrictor* / D

ergotamine / *migraine-specific analgesic* / D

ergots / *for migraine headaches* / ***D***

ERT / estrogen replacement therapy

eructation / *belching*

ERYC / Eryc / erythromycin / D

Erycette pledgets / *topical antibiotic for acne* / D

EryDerm / *wash / 2% topical solution / antibiotic* / D

Erygel / *for acne* / D

Ery Ped / *macrolide antibiotic* / D

erysipelas/-oid / *cellulitis of dermal lymphatics / usually from strep infection*

Ery-Tab / *macrolide antibiotic* / D

erythema / *warmth / effusion*

erythema annulare (Derm) / *red skin with rounded lesions*

erythema chronicum migrans (Derm) / *lesion formed from tick bite / typical skin lesion of Lyme disease*

erythema multiforme / (pronounced "multi-formee")

erythema nodosum (Derm)

erythematosus / *pertaining to erythema*

erythro-, eryth- / *red / color / red blood cells*

Erythrocin / erythromycin / *antibiotic* / D

erythrocytosis / *increased numbers of red blood cells*

Additional Entries

____

____

____

____

erythroid / *reddish in color*
erythropoiesis/-poietin / *substance secreted by the kidney*
eschar / *crust or slough that develops on burned skin*
Escherichia coli / E. coli / *coliform bacteria*
eschew / *to shun, as unworthy*
escutcheon / *pubic hair*
Esgic / *analgesic* / *sedative* / D
Esidrix / *diuretic* / *antihypertensive* / D
-esis / *condition* / *action* / *process* / *producing* / e.g., gen**esis**
Eskalith / *antipsychotic* / D
esophageal carcinoma
esophagitis / *inflammation of the esophagus*
esophagogastric
esophagogastroduodenoscopy
esophagram / esophagogram
esophagus, Nutcracker / *motility disorder with strong peristaltic contractions by the esophagus*
esotropia (Oph) / *cross-eyed*
ESR / erythrocyte sedimentation rate / T
essential / *hypertension* / *occurring without discoverable organic cause*
esterase / *generic term for certain enzymes*
esthesia, **-esthesia, -esthesio** / *sensation* / *feeling* / *consciousness* / *perception*
Estinyl / *hormone for estrogen replacement therapy (ERT) or inoperable breast or prostatic cancer* / D
Estrace / estradiol / *estrogen replacement for postmenopausal disorders* / *antineoplastic* / D
Estraderm / estradiol / *transdermal patch* / *estrogen replacement therapy (ERT) for menopausal disorders* / D
Estranyl / D

Additional Entries

Estratab / *estrogen replacement therapy (ERT)* / *for meno-pausal vasomotor symptoms* / D

Estratest / *estrogen/androgen* / D

Estrovis / *hormone replacement therapy* / D

ET / enterostomal therapy/therapist

ethacrynic acid / *diuretic* / D

ethambutol / *bacteriostatic* / *primary tuberculostatic* / D

Ethamolin / *ethanolamine oleate* / D

Ethiflex / *synthetic suture material*

Ethilon suture / 5-0 Ethilon suture

ethinyl / estradiol / D

ethmoid (Ortho) / *resembling a sieve* / *pertaining to the ethmoid bone*

E

Ethmozine / *antiarrhythmic* / D

etidronate / *calcium regulator* / D

etidronate therapy

etiology / *cause of condition*

E to A changes

ETOH abuse / ethyl alcohol abuse

etopóside / *antineoplastic* / D

Etrafon / *antipsychotic* / D

ETT / exercise treadmill test

eu- / *good* / *well* / (opposite of **dys-, caco-**)

Eucerin / *cream* / *moisturizer* / *emollient* / D

euglycemia / *normal blood glucose concentration*

Eulexin / flutamide (Chemo) / *hormone used in treatment of metastatic prostate cancer* / D

eustachian tube (ENT)

eusthenia / *normal strength*

Euthroid (discontinued 1992) / *thyroid hormone therapy* / D

euthyroid/-ism / *normally functioning thyroid* / *"happy thyroid"*

Additional Entries

____

____

____

____

evanescent / *vanishing / passing away quickly / unstable / unfixed*
eventration / *protrusion of omentum or intestine through abdomi-
    nal wall*
eversion / *turned outward*
evulsed / *forcibly extracted*
Ewing sarcoma / *bone tumor*
exacerbate / *to make worse*
exanthem (Derm) / *skin rash*
excoriation / *scratch or abrasion of the skin /*
    e.g., neurotic e. / *repeated self-inflicted excoriation*
excrescence / *any abnormal outgrowth*
exercise MUGA / (exercise) multigated angiogram / T
exercise thallium / T
exo- / exterior / external / outward
exogenetic/-ous / *originating outside the organism*
exophoria / exodeviation (Oph) / *eye deviation outward*
exophthalmic/-mos (Oph) / *pertaining to prominent eyeballs*
exophytic/-yte / *growth outward from an epithelial surface*
exostosis / *bony growth*
expansile / *pertaining to expanding / capable of expanding*
expiratory excursions (Pulm)
expiratory sibilant (Pulm)
exstrophy / *congenital eversion of a hollow organ*
extensor / *a muscle*
exteriorize / *to expose a part temporarily during surgery*
exteroception (Neuro)
Extra-Strength Tylenol / D [OTC]
extracorporeal / *outside the body*
extramedullary / *occurring outside the medulla oblongata*
extrapyramidal / *outside the pyramidal tracts*
extrasystoles / *premature contractions of the heart*

Additional Entries

____

____

____

____

extravasation / *discharge or escape of blood from a vessel into the tissues*

extrude / *to push out of a normal position or situation*

extubate/-ed / *to remove a tube from an orifice*

exudate/-tive / *a fluid that exudes out of body tissue or its capillaries, usually as a result of inflammation*

-e / *means of* / *instrument for* / e.g., telescop**e**

eyegrounds (Oph)

E

Additional Entries

FAC chemotherapy / 5FU, ADRIA, Cytoxan chemotherapy
facet / *smooth area on bone or other solid structure*
    e.g., f. arthritis; f. syndrome
facies / (pl.) facies / *face / surface / expression*
factor VIII (Hemo) / *hemophiliac treatment*
Fahrenheit / F.
fallopian tube(s) (Gyn)
familial / *family tendency to experience a medical
    condition(s)* / e.g., f. nephritis (Uro)
famotidine / Pepcid / *treatment of gastrointestinal ulcers* / D
Famvir / *for acute herpes zoster and genital herpes* / D
Fannenstiel...**NO!** (see "Pfannenstiel")
Fansidar / *antimalarial* / D
fascia/-ias / (pl.) fasciae, fascias / *fibrous covering over muscles*
    e.g., antebrachial f. / *wrist*; f. lata / *thigh*
fascial herniation
fasciculation / (pronounced "fasi-kul-ation") / *muscle contraction*
fasciitis, plantar / *feet*
fasciotomy
Fastin / *amphetamine-type anorectic / diet pill* / D
fatigability/-able
fatiguing
fat pad signs
FBS / fasting blood sugar / T
fecund / *fertile*
FEF / forced expiratory flow / T
Feingold diet
felbamate / Felbatol / *antiepileptic* / D
Feldene / piroxicam/ *nonsteroidal anti-inflammatory* / D
felodipine / Plendil / *for angina and hypertension* / D
Fem-Fem / *bypass graft*

F

Additional Entries
____
____
____
____

femoral / *femur or thigh*
femoropopliteal (Ortho) / *knee*
Femstat (discontinued 1995) / *vaginal cream* / *antifungal* / D
femur (Ortho) / *thigh bone*
Fenesin / guiafenesin / *expectorant* / D
fenfluramine / *anorexiant* / *central nervous system (CNS) depressant* / D
fenoprofen / Nalfon / *nonsteroidal anti-inflammatory* / D
fentanyl / Fentanyl / *analgesic* / *narcotic* / *anesthetic* / D
Feosol / *hematinic* / *iron supplement* / D
Fergon / *hematinic* / *antianemic* / *iron supplement* / D
Fergon-grains 5
ferritin / *level—iron protein complex* / T
Ferro-Sequels / *hematinic* / *iron supplement* / D
ferrous gluconate / *hematinic* / *iron supplement* / D
ferrous sulfate / *hematinic* / *iron supplement* / D
$FeSO_4$ / Ferrosulfate / *iron sulfate*
fetoprotein (see "alpha-fetoprotein")
FEV_1 / forced expiratory volume in one second / T
   also ... PFT / pulmonary function test / T
FFS / flexible fiberoptic sigmoidoscopy
Fiberall / *bulk laxative* / *antidiarrheal* / D
FiberCon / *bulk laxative* / *antidiarrheal* / D
fiberoptic proctosigmoidoscopy
fibrillation (Cardio) / *very rapid contractions or twitching of heart
   muscle*
fibrin / *elastic filamentlike protein*
fibrin demarcation
fibrinogen / *globulin of blood plasma converted into fibrin*
fibroadenoma / *benign tumor of the breast*
fibroadipose / *both fibrous and fatty tissue*
fibrochondroma / *tumor of fibrous tissue and cartilage*

Additional Entries

____

____

____

____

fibrocystic / *cystic spaces accompanied by an overgrowth of fibrous tissue*
fibrocystocytoma / *benign tumor*
fibromata / *plural of fibroma*
fibrositis / fibrositic / *muscular rheumatism*
fibrotic streaks
fidgety
filling defect / *on colon x-ray*
filtrum ventriculi / *pertaining to larynx*
fine needle aspiration
finger breadth
finger-to-nose and rapid alternating movements, past-pointing
Finkelstein feeding / *of infants*
Fioricet / *analgesic* / *sedative* / D
Fiorinal / *analgesic* / *anti-inflammatory* / *sedative* / D
fissura in ano / *anal fissure*
fist percussis / *fist moderately thumps area to be tested*
fistulogram
fistulous / *abnormal passage between two internal organs*
fixate and follow
fixateur/fixator, external
fixation device
Flagyl / metronidazole / *antibiotic* / *antiprotozoal* / *amebicide* / D
flatulence / flatus / *gastrointestinal gas or air*
flaxseed / linseed
flecainide / *antiarrhythmic* / D
flecks of calcium
Fleet Phospho-Soda / *buffered saline laxative*
Flex-all / *pain gel* / D [OTC]
Flexeril / *skeletal muscle relaxant* / D

F

Additional Entries

____
____
____
____

flexible fiberoptic sigmoidoscopy / flex sig
flexible torticollis / *neck twist*
flexion / *bending or flexing*
flexor / *muscle used to flex a joint*
flexor carpi radialis
flex sig / flexible fiberoptic sigmoidoscopy
flexure / *bent portion*
flip test / *ankle jerk*
Flonase nasal spray / *steroidal anti-inflammatory* / D
Florical / *calcium supplement* / D
florid / *bright red color*
Florinef / *for adrenocortical insufficiency in Addison disease* / D
Florone cream 0.05% / *for dermatitis* / D
Flovent inhaler / *corticosteroidal antiasthmatic* / D
flow tract (Cardiol) / *left ventricular*
Floxin / floxacillin and ofloxacin / *broad-spectrum antibiotic* / D
fluconazole / *broad-spectrum systemic fungistatic* / D
fluctuance / *varying levels* / *wavelike motion on palpation due to
    liquid content*
fludarabine / Fludara (Chemo) / D
fluid wave
Flumadine / rimantadine hydrochloride / *antiviral* / *for flu virus* / D
flumazenil / Romazicon / *antidote* / D
Fluocinonide / Lidex cream / *for relief of pain* / D
fluorescein (Oph) / *eye drops*
5-fluorouracil / 5-FU (Chemo)
fluoroquinolones
fluoroscopy / *x-rays under a fluoroscope*
Fluothane / *inhalation general anesthetic* / D
flurazepam / Dalmane / *anticonvulsant* / *sedative* / D
fluvastatin / Lescol / *cholesterol-lowering antihyperlipidemic* / D

Additional Entries

FNA / fine needle aspiration biopsy / e.g., FNA of node

foam cells / air cells

focal, symptoms / *chief center of a process*

foci / *plural of focus*

Fogarty catheter

folate / *a salt / ester of folic acid*

Foley catheter

follicle / *a sac or pouchlike depression or cavity*

folliculitis / *inflammation of a follicle*

Folstein Minimental / *mental test*

fomite / *agent which is not harmful in itself but may
    transmit infection*

foramen / *hole through bone or membranous structure*

foramen encroachment

foraminal / *opening*

foraminotomy / *an operation, usually to enlarge an opening*

Forestier disease / *of thoracic vertebral column*

forme fruste / *incomplete form*

-form / *shaped like / resembling* / denti**form**

fornix / (pl.) fornices / *an arch-shaped structure*

Fortaz / *intravenous antibiotic* / D

Fosamax / *for postmenopausal osteoporosis* / D

Fosfree / *vitamin/iron supplement* / D

fosinopril / Monopril / *antihypertensive / ACE inhibitor* / D

fossa / *trench or channel*

fourchette (Gyn) (pronounced "fur-shet") / (syn.) frenulum /
    vaginal / part of the labia minora

fracture, transverse

free thyroid / *thyroxine index* / T

Freiberg infarction

Fresinus machine / *for dialysis*

Additional Entries

---

fremitus / *vibration*
friable / *easily reduced to powder*
Friedrich ataxia / *in hereditary spinocerebellar disease*
frontal hemisphere
frozen with LN2 (liquid nitrogen)
Frykman-8 fracture
FSBS / finger stick blood sugar
FSH / follicle stimulating hormone (index) / T
5 FU / fluorouracil (Chemo)
Fuch dystrophy / *syndrome*
FUDS / fluorourodynamic study
fulguration / *cauterization* / *destruction of tissue with high-frequency electric current*
full and equal without bruits
fulminant / *happening suddenly, with great severity*
Fulvicin / griseofulvin / *systemic antifungal* / D
fundoplication, Nissen / *to treat reflux esophagitis*
fundus / fundal / *bottom or base of anything* / *area farthest removed from mouth of an organ*
funduscopic / ophthalmoscopic
fungating / *to grow prolifically, like a fungus*
Fungizone / *topical antifungal* / D
Furadantin / nitrofurantoin / *urinary bacteriostatic* / D
furosemide / Lasix / *loop diuretic* / D
furuncle / *infection in a hair follicle* / *a boil*
furunculosis / *having multiple furuncles, often a chronic condition*
fusiform / *swelling*
fusion / *melting*
Futura / *wrist splints*
FVC / forced vital capacity / *test of pulmonary function*
FVD / fibrovascular tissue on disk

Additional Entries

____

____

____

____

gabapentin / Neurontin / *anticonvulsant* / D

gadolinium / *element used in magnetic resonance imaging (MRI)*

galactorrhea (Gyn) / *excessive or spontaneous flow of milk irrespective of nursing*

gallbladder

gallium scan / T

gamma GT / glutamyl transferase

gammopathy / *disturbance in immunoglobulin synthesis*

ganglion / *knotlike mass*

Gantrisin / *ophthalmic bacteriostatic* / D

gap, anion / *used in evaluation of acid-base disorders*

Garamycin Ophthalmic / *antibiotic* / D

Gardnerella (Gyn) / *bacteria found in vaginitis*

Garré disease / osteomyelitis

GASA (Ortho) / growth-adjusted sonographic age

Gas-X / *chewable antiflatulent* / D [OTC]

gaseous

gastr-, gastro- / *stomach* / *abdomen*

gastralgia / *stomach ache*

gastric II diet

gastric outlet obstruction (GI)

gastrins / *hormones* (GI)

gastritis, antral (GI)

gastrocnemius / *muscle* / *knee*

gastroesophageal (GI)

Gastrografin / *radiological contrast media*

gastrojejunostomy / *creating a connection between stomach and jejunum*

gastroparesis (GI) / *minimal gastroparalysis*

gastroscopy

Additional Entries

____

____

____

____

gaited / *manner of walking*
gated / *opening and closing channel*
Gaucher disease / *splenomegaly (enlarged spleen)*
gauge
Gaviscon / *antacid* / D [OTC]
Gel-Cam ointment
gel cast (Ortho)
gemfibrozil / *antihyperlipoproteinemic* / D
gen- / *original* / *production* / e.g., **gen**esis
-gen / *that which is produced* / e.g., patho**gen** / hydro**gen**
genit- / *reproduction* / *the organs of reproduction* / e.g., **genit**alia
genitalia / *organs of reproduction*
genitourinary / *reproductive and urinary systems*
Genora / *monophasic oral contraceptive* / D
Genprobe (Gyn) / *for gonorrhea culture (GC) and Chlamydia* / T
gentamicin / *bacterial antibiotic* / D
genu valgus / *knock knee*
genu varum / *bowleg*
Geocillin / *for urinary tract infection or prostatitis* / D
geographic tongue / *benign migratory glossitis*
ger-, **geron-**, **geronto-** / *old* / *old person* / *old age* /
    e.g., **gero**derma, **geronto**therapy
geri chair (Gerontology)
geroderma / *atrophic skin of the aged* / *any condition in which skin*
    is thin and wrinkled like that of old people
gerontotherapy / geriatric therapy / *treatment of disease in the aged*
Gesell (Peds)
gestational diabetes / *the diabetes of pregnancy*
GGT / gamma glutamyl transferase / T
Ghon complex / *primary lesion, tubercle*
GI / gastrointestinal

Additional Entries

Giardia Blastocystis Hominis / *intestinal parasite*
giardiasis / *intestinal infection*
gibbus (n.) / gibbous (adj.) / *deformity* / *a hump*
GI cocktail
Gilbert syndrome
gingiv-, gingivo- / *the gums*
gingivitis / *inflammation of the gums*
ginkgo supplement
GITS / glipizide / *antidiabetic* / D
glabella / *prominence above root of nose* / *projecting point of forehead*
glans / L. acorn / *acorn-shaped structure* / e.g., g. clitoris; g. penis
glans area
glaucoma (Oph) / *increase in intraocular pressure causing pathological changes in vision*
glenohumeral / *joints*
gliamilide / *antidiabetic* / D
glioblastoma multiforme / *primary tumor of the brain*
glioma / *neoplasms of the brain and spinal cord*
glipizide GITS / g. glutathione-insulin transhydrogenase / *antidiabetic* / D
Glisson capsule / *fibrous capsule of the liver*
global development / *occurring everywhere*
globulin / *proteins*
globus hystericus / *sensation of a lump in the throat*
glomerulonephritis / *inflammation in the kidney*
glomerulus/-uli / *cluster of blood vessels or nerve fibers in the kidney*
gloss-, glossa-, glosso- / *tongue*
glossal / *lingual*

G

Additional Entries

glossitis / *inflammation of the tongue*
glucagon / *for diabetes* / D
glucagonoma / *a sometimes malignant tumor of pancreatic islets*
Glucerna / *therapy for abnormal glucose tolerance* / D
glucocorticoid
glucometer strips / *diagnostic aid for blood glucose*
Glucophage / *biguanide antidiabetic* / D
glucosuria / *sugar in the urine*
Glucotrol / *sulfonylurea-type antidiabetic* / D
gluteal / *the buttocks*
glyburide / *antidiabetic* / D
glycosylated/-ion / *hemoglobin test* / T
glycosuria / *older variant of the word "glucose"* / *in the urine*
Glynase PresTabs / *for diabetes* / D
gm / gram
gm/dl / grams per deciliter
Gohn complex...**NO!** (see "Ghon complex")
goiter / *enlargement of the thyroid gland*
    colloid g. / *goiter is large, soft, and greatly distended*
    multinodular g. / *thyroid contains circumscribed nodules*
gold treatment / *for arthritis*
Goldman elevator
GoLYTELY / *powder* / *for bowel cleansing* / D
gonococcus (GC) / gonococcal / gonococci / *organism that causes gonorrhea*
gonorrhea / *sexually transmitted infection*
Goody's powders / *analgesic* / *anti-inflammatory* / *for headaches* / D
Gore-Tex / *suture and graft material*
Gottron's nodule / *in dermatomyositis*
Gottschalk Nasostat / *rubber cannula used to stop nosebleeds*
G1P1AB0 / one pregnancy, one child, no abortions

Additional Entries

G7P6AB1 / seven pregnancies, six children, one abortion

gradatim (L.) / *gradually* / *by degrees*

gradient

-gram / *write* / *record* / *draw* / *printed record by an instrument* / e.g., tele**gram;** electrocardio**gram**

gram stain

granular casts / *made up of granules or grains*

Granulex / *topical spray for wound debridement* / D

granulocytopenia / agranulocytosis

granuloma / *nodular inflammatory lesions, usually small*

granuloma annulare (Derm) / *granulomatous disease of the dermis*

granulomatous / *having granules*

granulopoiesis / *the formation of granulocytes*

graphesthesia / *ability to recognize figures or numbers when written on the skin with a dull-pointed object*

Graves disease / *disorder of the thyroid*

gravida (Gyn) / *pregnant woman* / *written number preceding g. or number after g. indicates number of pregnancies* / e.g., primigravida *(first pregnancy);* gravida II *(second pregnancy)*

grayish

Greenfield filter / Kim-Ray Greenfield / *used in autosomal recessive disorder (leukodystrophy)*

Grifulvin V / griseofulvin / *systemic antifungal* / D

grimacing / *facial contortion expressing pain, contempt or disgust*

Grisactin / *antifungal* / D

Griseofulvin / *antifungal* / D

Gris-PEG / griseofulvin / *antifungal* /D

grumose / grumous / *thick and lumpy*

GU / genitourinary

guaiac / *reagent*

Additional Entries

____

____

____

____

Guaifed / *decongestant* / *expectorant* / D
guaifenesin / glycerol guaiacolate / *expectorant* / D
Guaitab / *decongestant* / *expectorant* / D
Guaituss / *for cough* / D
guarding / *muscle spasm* / *deliberate muscle tension to protect tender or injured area*
Guillain-Barré syndrome (pronounced "gee-yahn bah-ray") / *acute febrile polyneuritis*
gustatory / *pertaining to taste or the sense of taste*
guttate / *lesions shaped like a drop* / *seen in psoriasis*
gyn, Gyn, GYN / gynecology / *study of women's diseases*
gynecologic
gynecomastia / *male breast development*
Gyne-Lotrimin / D

Additional Entries

____

____

____

____

Habitrol / *transdermal patch* / *for nicotine withdrawal* / D
habitus / *physical characteristics of a person* /
    e.g., gracile h. / *small stature* / *frail* / *underweight*
Haglund disorder / Haglund disease / *callused heels*
Halcion / *sleep inducing drug* / D
Haldol / *antipsychotic* / *for Tourette syndrome* / D
Halfprin / *anti-inflammatory* / *antirheumatic* / D
hallux valgus / *angulation of great toes away from midline*
    of a body or toward the other toes
hallux varus / *great toes angled away from other toes or*
    toward midline of the body
halo nevi
Halog cream / *topical corticosteroid anti-inflammatory* / D
haloperidol / *antidyskinetic* / *antipsychotic* / *for Tourette*
    disease / D
Halotex lotion / *topical antifungal* / D
Halsted inguinal herniorrhaphy / *operation*
hamartoma / *benign tumor* / *overgrowth of cells*
Hapad / *foot lift*
haptoglobin / *plasma glycoprotein*
Harada disease (Oph)
harasses
Harrington rods (Ortho) / *scoliosis*
Hashimoto thyroid / *thyroiditis*
haustral markings / *saccules that resemble a water wheel*
HAV / hepatitis A virus
H2 blocker
HBV / hepatitis B virus
hCG / beta-HCG / *menses check* / *pregnancy test* / T
hCG serum / human chorionic gonadotropin s. / *pregnancy test* / T
HCTZ / hydrochlorothiazide / *for blood pressure control* / D

Additional Entries

____
____
____
____

HDL / high-density lipoproteins / *"the good cholesterol"*
Heberden nodes / *hard nodules, usually distal interphalangeal joints of fingers / in osteoarthritis*
heel cord stretching exercises
HEENT / head, eyes, ears, nose (and) throat / *portion of physical examination*
Heimlich maneuver / *dislodge food or other material from the throat of a choking victim*
Helicobacter pylori (GI) / *A genus of bacteria associated with ulcers*
heliotrope rash / *pale purple rash*
heloma durum / *hard corn*
heloma molle / *soft corn*
hem- (at) - / *blood ("h" dropped when used in middle of word)*
  -emia / condition of blood / e.g., cyan**em**ia
hemangioendothelioma
hemangioma / *proliferation of blood vessels / congenital anomaly*
hemarthrosis / *blood in a joint*
hematemesis / *vomiting blood*
hematochezia / (pronounced "hemato-keesia")
hematocrit / *determination of the volume of packed red cells in the blood* / T
hematogenous spread
hematospermia / *blood in seminal fluid*
hematostaxis / *spontaneous bleeding due to disease of blood*
hematuria / *blood in urine*
heme-negative / *no blood in stool*
hemi- / *one-half / semi / part of*
hemianopsia/-opia (Oph) / *loss of vision of one half visual field*
hemiatrophy / *atrophy of one half or part of an organ*
hemicolectomy / *removal of half of the colon*
hemidiaphragm

Additional Entries

____

____

____

____

hemimelia / *developmental absence of all or part of the distal half of a limb*
hemiparesis/-etic / *weakness on one side of body*
hemiplegia / *paralysis on one side of body*
hemithorax / *one side of thorax*
Hemoccult / *test for blood in stool* / T
hemochromatosis / *abnormal iron metabolism*
hemodialysis / *removal of waste products from blood* / *substitute for kidneys*
hemodynamic/-ally / *pertaining to blood circulation*
hemoglobin A_{1c}
hemolytic
Hemophilus hemolyticus / *bacterium*
Hemophilus influenzae meningitis / *bacterium*
hemopoietic / hematopoietic
hemoptysis / *expectoration (spitting) of blood*
hemorrhage/-agic / *abnormal discharge of blood*
hemorrhoidectomy / *excision of hemorrhoids*
hemosiderin / *storage form of iron*
hemosiderosis / *increase in tissue iron stores*
hemostat / *agent that stops blood flow from vessels*
hemotympanum / *a hemorrhagic exudation into the middle ear*
heparin / *anticoagulant* / *blood thinner* / D
hepat-, hepatico-, hepato- / *the liver*
hepatic flexure
hepatitis B / *inflammation of the liver*
hepatocellular
hepatosplenomegaly / *enlargement of the liver and the spleen*
Heptavax / *immunization*
herald patch (Derm) / *the solitary lesion preceding general eruption in pityriasis rosea*

H

Additional Entries

---

hernia / e.g., diaphragmatic h.; nonincarcerated h.; inguinal h.
herniation
herniorrhaphy/-ies
herpes genitalis / genital herpes
herpes labialis
herpes simplex virus / HSV
herpes zoster
herpetic whitlow / *lesion*
Hertz frequencies
hexachlorophene / *topical anti-infective* / D
hiatal hernia
HGB / Hgb / hemoglobin
H&H / hematocrit and hemoglobin (hemogram)
5-HIAA / (5) hydroxyindoleacetic acid
Hib / HIB / Haemophilus influenzae type b (vaccine)
Hibiclens / *skin cleanser* / *broad-spectrum antimicrobial, germi-
    cidal prep* / D
Hickman catheter
HIDA scan / hepatic 2,6-dimethyliminodiacetic acid (scan) /
    (pronounced "hyda")
hidradenitis suppurativa / *chronic presence of pus in certain
    sweat glands*
hidro-, hidr- / *sweat* / *sweat glands*
hidrosis / *sweating*
high-dose
high power field
hilar / *pertaining to the depression or pit at the part of an organ
    where the vessels and nerves enter*
hemicolectomy
hilum / *depression or pit at the part of an organ where the vessels
    and nerves enter*

Additional Entries

____

____

____

____

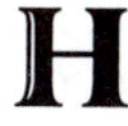

hippuria / *hippuric acid in urine*
hippuran / I-131 *labeled sodium*
Hirschsprung disease / *congenital megacolon*
hirsutism / *hairiness*
Hismanal / *nonsedating antihistamine* / D
hist-, histo- / *tissue*
histiocytic
Histalet / *decongestant* / *antihistamine* / D
histolytic
histopathologic
histoplasmosis (Pulm) / *fungal infection of the lungs*
HIV / human immunodeficiency virus
HIV and RPR (Cardio) /   . . . rapid plasma reagin
hMG / human menopausal gonadotropin
HMG CoA reductase / *inhibitor*
HMO / health maintenance organization
H/O / h/o / history of
Hodgkin disease
holosystolic murmur (Cardio)
Holter monitor (Cardio)
Homan sign / *in leg thrombosis, forced dorsiflexion of foot causes
   pain behind knee*
homogeneous / *uniform quality throughout*
homogenous / *structural similarity because of descent from a
   common ancestor*
homonymous / *the same name or expressed in same terms*
hordeolum (Oph) / *inflammation of eyelid gland* / *sty/stye*
Horner syndrome / *sinking of eyeball* / *ptosis of upper eyelid*
host disease
H&P / history and physical
HPV / human papilloma virus

Additional Entries

____
____
____
____

HR / heart rate
HS / h.s. / (L. *hora somni*) / *on retiring* / *at bedtime*
   e.g., h.s. antacids; h.s. Maalox
HSV / herpes simplex virus
HTLV / human T-cell lymphotropic virus
HTLV-III
H. pylori / Helicobacter pylori / *bacterium causing ulcers*
HTV / herpes-type virus
Huber opponensplasty
Humalog / *injection* / *for diabetes* / D
humectant / *a moisturizer*
humerus/-i (Ortho) / *arm bone*
Humibid / *antitussive* / *expectorant* / D
humoral immune deficiency
Humulin N / *subcutaneous injection* / *antidiabetic* / D
Hunter canal / *operation*
Huntington chorea / *mental deterioration terminating in dementia*
Hurthle cell tumor / *found in thyroid gland*
HX / history
hyaline / *glassy transparent membrane*
hyalinosis / *hyaline degeneration*
hyaluronic acid (Oph) / *ophthalmic surgical aid*
Hycodan / *narcotic antitussive* / D
Hycomine / *pediatric narcotic antitussive* / D
hydatid cyst / *cystlike structure*
Hydergine / *sublingual* / *for age-related mental capacity decline* / D
hydralazine / *antihypertensive* / *vasodilator* / D
Hydrea / *antineoplastic* / *for melanoma* / D
hydro- / **hydr-** / *water* / *fluid accumulated in body part*
   hidro- / **hidr-** / *sweat gland* / *sweat gland*
   hygro- / **hygr-** / *moisture* / *humidity*

Additional Entries

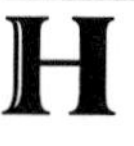

hydrocephalus / *enlarged head due to accumulation of cerebrospinal fluid in the ventricles of the brain*

hydrocele / *collection of fluid in testicle or spermatic cord*

hydrochlorothiazide / HCTZ / *diuretic / antihypertensive* / D

hydrocodone / *antitussive* / D

hydrocortisone / *corticosteroid* / D

HydroDIURIL / *diuretic / antihypertensive* / D

hydromorphone / *narcotic / analgesic* / D

hydronephrosis / *distention of the pelvis and kidneys with urine*

Hydropres / *antihypertensive* / D

hydrops / *edema / excessive accumulation of fluid in body*

hydrosalpinx / *collection of watery fluid in uterine tube / endstage of pyosalpinx*

hydroxyurea / Hydrea / *antineoplastic* / D

hydroxyzine / *anxiolytic / antihistamine* / D

hyfrecated / Hyfrecator / *skin tags*

hygroma (hydroma) / *watery cyst*

Hygroton / *diuretic / antihypertensive* / D

Hymenoptera / *bees / wasps / ants*

hyoid / *shaped like a "U" or a "V"* / e.g., h. bone / *in throat*

hyoscyamine / *anticholinergic* / D

hyp-, hyper- / *above / more than normal / excessive*

hyperacusis / *abnormally acute hearing*

hyperadrenergic / *secreting excessive epinephrine or related substances*

hyperalbuminemia / proteinemia / *albumin in the blood*

hyperaldosteronism / *secretion of excessive aldosterone hormone*

hyperalimentation / *more than basic nutrient requirements*

hyperammonemia / *excessive amount of ammonia in the blood*

hyperbaric oxygen / *under greater than atmospheric pressure*

Additional Entries

---

hypercalcemia / *an excess of calcium in the blood*

hypercalciuria/-ic / *excessive excretion of calcium salts in urine*

hypercarotenemia / *excessive carotene in the blood*

hypercellularity / *abnormal increase in the number of cells present, as in bone marrow*

hyperchloremic / *severe iron deficiency anemia*

hypercholesterolemia / *extreme levels of cholesterol in blood*

hypercoagulable / *excessive clotting*

hyperemic/-emia / *excessive blood in a body part / engorgement*

hyperemesis gravidarum (Gyn) / *excessive vomiting during pregnancy*

hyperesthesia / *excessive sensitivity*

hyperkalemia / *abnormally high levels of potassium in blood*

hyperinsulinemic / *excessive levels of insulin in blood*

hyperlipemia / hyperlipidemia / *excessive lipids in blood*

hyperlipidemia, type IV

hyperlucency / *increased radiolucency*

hypermenorrhea / *excessive uterine bleeding / menorrhagia*

hypernatremia / *excessive amount of sodium in the blood*

hyperosmolar / *excessive increase in osmolar concentration*

hyperostosis (Ortho) / *hypertrophy of bone*
    e.g., ankylosing h. / *diffuse idiopathic skeletal hyperostosis*

hyperparathyroidism / *excessive parathyroid hormone*

hyperpigmentation / *increase in skin pigmentation*

hyperplasia/-tic / *increase in cells in tissue or organ*

hyperprolactinemia / *abnormally high levels of prolactin in blood*

hyperpyrexia / *elevated body temperature / body temperature above 106° (41.1° C.) / produced by physical agents such as hot baths*

hyperreflexia / *exaggeration of deep tendon reflexes*

hyperresonance / *extreme resonance upon percussion of body area*

Additional Entries

____

____

____

____

hyperserotonergic / *abnormal amounts of serotonin in blood*

H

hypersomnia/-ence / *excessively long periods of sleep*

hypersplenism / *abnormal rate at which spleen removes cellular components of blood*

hypertension / *abnormally high blood pressure*

hyperthyroidism / *excessive production of thyroid hormones, marked by goiter*

hypertonus / *increased resistance of muscle to passive stretching*

hypertriglyceridemia / *elevated levels of triglycerides in the blood*

hypertrophic spurring / *overgrowth of projections from a bone*

hypertrophy / *overall increase in bulk or size of a body part or organ, not due to tumor*

hyperuricemia / *increased concentrations of uric acid in the blood*

hypervolemia / *excessive volume of blood*

hypha/-ae / *tubular cell typical of fungi*

hyphal / *pertaining to hypha*

hypnagogic / hypnotic / *pertaining to the hypnoticlike state preceding sleep / inducing sleep / induced by sleep*

hypo- / *underneath / deficient / below normal*

hypoadrenergic state / *undersecretion of epinephrine*

hypoalbuminemia / *abnormally low albumin content in the blood*

hypoattenuation / *on ultrasound imaging studies, producing less strong a signal, showing tumors*

hypocalcemia / *excessivily low levels of calcium in blood*

hypocitruria / *abnormally low levels of citrate in urine*

hypocycloidal / *mood swings*

hypoeccrisis/ *smaller amounts of excreted waste matter*

hypoechoic / *weaker and fewer echoes in ultrasound image area*

Additional Entries

____

____

____

____

hypoesthesia / hypesthesia / *lessening sensitivity to stimulation*

hypoestrogenic / *underproduction of estrogen*

hypogastrium / *situated inferior to the stomach*

hypogonadotropic / *abnormal gonadal development and/or function*

hypokalemia / *abnormally low levels of potassium in the blood*

hypokinesis / *decrease in movement / no movement*

hypomagnesemia / *excessively low levels of magnesium in the blood*

hyponatremia / *abnormally low levels of sodium in the blood*

hypophysectomy / *surgical removal of the pituitary gland*

hypoplastic / *undeveloped tissue or organ*

hypopnea / *abnormally shallow breathing / slow breathing*

hyporeflexia / *weakened reflexes*

hypothalamic amenorrhea / *amenorrhea due to the hypothalamus*

hypothenar / *pertaining to the palm* / e.g., h. eminence

hypothyroidism / *decreased levels of thyroid*

hypouricemia / *abnormally low levels of uric acid in the blood*

hypovolemia / *low quantity of blood in body*

hypoxemia/-emic / *abnormally low oxygenation of arterial blood*

hyster- / *womb*

hysterectomy (Gyn) / *surgical removal of uterus*

hysterosalpingogram/-graphy (Gyn) / *record of surgical removal of uterus and one or both uterine tubes*

hysteroscopy (Gyn) / *visual examination of uterine cavity using scope*

Hytone / hydrocortisone / *cream / topical corticosteroid*

Hytrin / terazosin / *antihypertensive / treatment for benign prostatic hyperplasia / D*

Hyzaar / losartan and hydrochlorothiazide / *antihypertensive / diuretic / D*

Additional Entries

I&A / I/A / irrigation and aspiration
IABC (Cardio) / intra-aortic balloon catheter
-iasis / *condition* / *presence of* / *state of* / *disease* /
    e.g., lith**iasis**
-a / *a disease* / *unhealthy condition* / e.g., amnesi**a**
iatrogenic / *response, usually unfavorable, to medical or
    surgical treatment*
IBC / iron binding capacity
Iberet-500 / *filmtabs* / *hematinic* / D
IBS / irritable bowel syndrome
ibuprofen / *antiarthritic* / *nonsteroidal* / *anti-inflammatory
    analgesic* / D
-ical / *pertaining to* / e.g., pract**ical**
ichthyo-/-oid / *fish*
ichthyosis/-otic / *skin disorder* / *"fish" skin* / *noninflammatory
    scaling*
-ic / **-ics** / *organized knowledge of science or art* / *study of* /
    e.g., mathemat**ics**; anesthet**ics**
-ic / *pertaining to* / e.g., hero**ic**
ictal / *pertaining to or caused by a stroke or acute epileptic seizure*
icterus/-ic / (syn.) jaundice
ICU / intensive care unit
Icy Hot / *balm* / *counterirritant*
ID / identification
I&D / incision and drainage
ideation / idea
-ide / *chemical compound ending* / e.g., brom**ide**; cyan**ide**
idio- / *private* / *peculiar to* / *unique*
idiopathic/-pathy / agnogenic / *a disease of unknown origin or
    etiology*
ifosfamide / *ankylating antineoplastic* / D

Additional Entries

____

____

____

____

Ig / immunoglobulin (e.g., IgA, IgG, IgM antibodies)

Il-2 / interleukin-2 / *recombinant*

il**eac** / ileum (GI-GU) / *distal portion of small intestine, from jejunum to cecum*
   (compare to) ... il**iac** (Ortho) / *upper area of hip bone*

ileal loop

ileectomy / *excision of the ileum*

ileo- / *the ileum / bottom of the small intestine*

ileocecal / *pertaining to both ileum and cecum*

ileoproctostomy / *creating a link between ileum and rectum*

ileorectal

ileostomy / *creating a fistula through which the ileum empties directly to the outside of the body*

ileum / *bottom part of the small intestine*

ileus / *bowel obstruction*

iliac crest / *upper area of hip bone*

iliofemoral / *pertaining to both the ilium and the femur*

ilioinguinal / *pertaining to both the iliac area and the groin*

iliopsoas / *muscle that flexes thigh or trunk*

iliotibial / *pertaining to both the ilium and the tibia* / e.g., i. band

ilium/-ia / *hipbone*

Ilotycin ointment / *ophthalmic antibiotic* / D

IM / intramuscularly

Imdur / *angina preventative* / D

Imferon (discontinued) / *intramuscular injection / antianemic* / D

imipramine / *tricyclic antidepressant* / D

Imitrex / *antimigraine* / D

immotile cilia syndrome / *primary ciliary dyskinesia* / D

immune thrombocytopenia / *decreased number of blood platelets*

immunoelectrophoresis / *distinct elliptical precipitant arc for a protein, detectable by the antisera*

Additional Entries

____

____

____

____

immunofluorescence / *antibody labeled with a fluorescent dye*

immunoglobulin / *glycoproteins that function as antibodies*

immunologic / *pertaining to immune phenomena*

immunosuppressive / *prevention or diminution of the immune response*

Imodium / *antidiarrheal* / D

impedance / *total opposition to flow*

impetiginization/-inous (Derm) / *development of impetigo on skin with another skin disease*

impetigo (Derm) / *contagious skin disease*

Imuran / *immunosuppressant for organ transplantation* / D

in- / *not* / *in* / *within* / *inside* / e.g., **in**organic; **in**clusion

-in / *organic compounds* / e.g., melan**in**

Inapsine / *intravenous or intramuscular general anesthetic* / D

incarcerated / *confined* / *imprisoned* / *trapped*

incentive spirometry / *to blow hard into spirometer after surgery to keep lungs open*

incipient / *beginning to exist* / *appear* / *initial*

incoherent / *not coherent*

incontinence / *inability to control discharge of urine or feces*

incus necrosis (ENT) / *cell death of anvil of the ear*

indapamide / Lozol / *antihypertensive* / D

Inderal / *antianginal* / *antihypertensive* / *migraine preventative* / D

Inderide / *antihypertensive* / D

index/-ices / index finger / *a guide* / *standard* / *ratio*

indices / *plural of index*

indirect inguinal hernia / *external or oblique hernia*

Indium scan / *blue metal* / *atomic number 49*

Indochron / *nonsteroidal anti-inflammatory* / D

Indocin SR / *nonsteroidal anti-inflammatory* / D

Additional Entries

---

indolent / *slow growing* / *inactive*
indomethacin / *nonsteroidal anti-inflammatory* / D
induration / *hardness*
Infanrix DtaP / *diphtheria and tetanus toxoid* / *vaccine for children up to age seven*
infero / *below*
inferobasal / *situated inferior to the base*
infiltrative ductal carcinoma (Onc) / *accumulation of abnormal substances in a cell or tissue*
inflammation / *injury to cells/tissue* / *marked by redness, heat, pain*
infra-areolar / *inferior to areola*
infraclavicular / subclavian
infrapatellar bursitis / *below patella*
infraspinatus / *muscle*
infundibulum / *funnel-shaped structure*
inguinal / *pertaining to the groin*
infraspinatus / *muscle*
INH / isonicotinic acid hydrazide (isoniazid) / D
inhalant
inhomogeneous / *not of uniform quality throughout*
initis / myositis / *inflammation of fibrous tissue*
innate / inborn
innocent heart murmur / *benign* / *not tending toward a fatal issue*
innocuous / *harmless*
innominate / *no name*
Inocor / amrinone lactate / *vasodilator* / *for congestive heart failure* / D
inoscopic/-opy / *microscopic examination*
INR / international normalized ratio / T
insalubrious / *unhealthful, especially in reference to climate*
insenescence / *process of growing old*

Additional Entries

____

____

____

____

in situ / *in place*

inspire / *inhale*

InspirEase / *portable inhalation device* / D

inspissation / *thickening or condensing secretions*

instillations / *drop by drop*

insudate / *fluid swelling within an arterial wall*

insulin / *pancreas secretion* / *hormone that regulates sugar metabolism*

insufflation / *to blow into* / *injection of gas or air into a body cavity* / *i.e., prior to laparoscopy, the abdomen is insufflated, inflated with carbon dioxide*

Intal inhaler / *bronchodilator for bronchial asthma* / D

inter- / *among* / *between*

interarticular / interarticularis (Ortho) / *between two joints or joint surfaces*

interbronchial

intercadent / *irregular in rhythm*

intercalary / *occurring between* / *interposed*

intercostal / *between ribs*

intercurrent / intervening / *a disease that occurs to a person who already has another ailment*

interferon / *antineoplastic* / D

interfollicular

intergluteal / *between the buttocks*

interleukin / *antineoplastic* / D

intermenstrual (Gyn) / *between menses* / *bleeding between menses*

interosseous (Ortho) / *between bones, as muscles and ligaments*

interphalangeal (Ortho) / *between finger or toe joints*

interscapular (Ortho) / *between scapulae* / *between shoulder blades*

interseptal / *between two walls*

interstitial fibrosis / *fibrous tissue within the cells*

Additional Entries

____

____

____

____

intertriginous (Derm) / *eczema on apposed skin surfaces, as under breasts*

intertrigo (Derm) / *dermatitis between folds of skin*

intertrochanteric (Ortho) / *between the two trochanters of the femur*

intervascular / *within blood vessels*

intervertebral iliotibial band

intra-abdominal / *within the abdomen*

intra-aortic balloon pump

intradermal / *within the dermis*

intradialytic hyperalimentation

intraductal / *occurring within the duct of a gland*

intraepithelial / *situated among the cells of the epithelium*

intramuscular / *into or within a muscle*

intraocular (Oph) / *within the eyeball*

intrasellar / *in a transverse depression over the sphenoid bone / wedge-shaped bone at the base of the skull*

intrauterine (Gyn) / *within the uterus*

intravenous / *within a vein*

intravesiceal / intravesical / *within the bladder*

intrinsic muscles / *situated on the inside*

introital / introitus / *entrance into canal or hollow organ / e.g., the vagina*

intromission / *placing one inside the other*

intubation / *to insert a tube into the larynx*

intussusception / *prolapse / of colorectal or mitral valve*

inure / *become accustomed to something difficult or painful*

involutional / *rolling back to normal size, as female organs after delivery / shriveling of organs and tissues with advancing age*

Iodamoeba butschlii

iodoform gauze / *powder / topical anti-infective, 96% iodine / soluble in chloroform and ether*

Additional Entries

---

iodoquinol / Yodoxin / *amebicide* / D
Ionamin / *anorexiant* / D
Ionil-T Plus / *shampoo* / *antiseborrheic* / *antibacterial* / D
ionized PTH calcium
iontophoresis / ionic medication
-ion / *action* / *condition resulting from action* / e.g., incis**ion**
Iopidine / *eye drops* / *antiglaucoma agent* / D
-ior / *more* / *toward* / e.g., inter**ior**
IPPB / intermittent positive pressure breathing
IPPD / PPD / purified protein derivative (of tuberculin) /
   tuberculosis skin test / T
IPPV / intermittent positive pressure ventilation
ipratropium bromide 0.025% solution / Atrovent /
   bronchodilator / D
ipsilateral / *on the same side*
iridectomy (Oph)
irides (Oph) / *plural of iris*
iridium wire / *made of very hard white metal, atomic number 77*
iris / (pl.) irides (Oph)
iritis (Oph) / *inflammation of the iris*
iron deficiency anemia
irradiation therapy
irritable bowel / *alternating diarrhea and constipation*
-is / *noun ending* / e.g., derm**is**
ischemia / *deficiency of blood in a part, as in heart muscle*
ischial / *part of the hip bone*
ischiorectal / *pertaining to the ischium and rectum*
ischium/-ia (Ortho) / *lower, back part of hip bone*
Ismo / isosorbide mononitrate / *angina preventative* / D
Isoclor / *decongestant* / *antihistamine* / D
isodense / *tissue with a radiopacity similar to that of adjacent tissue*

Additional Entries

____

____

____

____

isophane / *insulin* / D
isoproterenol inhaler / *bronchodilator* / D
Isoptin / *antihypertensive* / D
Isordil / *antianginal* / D
isometheptene / *for vascular headaches* / D
isoniazid / inh / *bactericidal* / *tuberculostatic* / D
isosorbide mononitrate / Ismo / *coronary vasodilator* / D
isotretinoin drug study / *keratolytic* / D
isradipine / DynaCirc / *antihypertensive* / D
-ist / *one who practices* / *does* / *is concerned with* / e.g., pharma**cist**
isthmus / *constriction joining two larger parts of an organ or other body structure*
-itis / inflammation of / e.g., nephr**itis**
itraconazole / *systemic antifungal* / D
IU/ml / microunits per milliliter
IUD / intrauterine device
-ium / *place* / *region* / *lining* / *covering tissue* / e.g., pod**ium**; epithel**ium**
IV / intravenously
IVP / intravenous pyelogram
IV push

Additional Entries

Jaboulay amputation / *amputation of the thigh and removal of the hip bone*

Jaboulay button / *two cylinders that are screwed together / for intestinal anastomosis without use of sutures*

jackscrew / *screw used in appliance to separate teeth or jaws*

jactatio / jactitation / *restless tossing of the head and body / seen in acute illness*

Jamar dynamometer / *device for measuring muscular strength*

Janeway lesion / *lesion on the palm / in subacute bacterial endocarditis*

jaundice / *liver disease / characterized by yellow-tinted skin*

jejun-, jejuno- / *pertaining to the jejunum / part of the small intestine*

jejunoileal (GI-GU) / *pertaining to the jejunum and the ileum*

jejunoileitis (GI-GU) / *inflammation of the jejunum and the ileum*

jejunostomy (GI-GU) / *surgical creation of a permanent opening from the abdominal wall into the jejunum*

jejunotomy / *incision into the jejunum*

jejunum (GI-GU) / *that portion of the small intestine between the duodenum and the ileum*

Jelco / *IV tubing / for cerumen impaction*

jelling

Jevity / *tube feeding*

Jheri chair

Jobst / *stockings*

JOD / JD / juvenile-onset diabetes

JODM / JDM / juvenile-onset diabetes mellitus

joint line

Additional Entries

____

____

____

____

joints
    carpometacarpal j. / thumb j.
    coccygeal j. / saccroccygeal j.
    cubital j. / elbow j.
    DIP / distal interphalangeal j. / fingers and toes
    intercarpal j. / carpal j. / wrist j.
    mandibular j. / temporomandibular j. / jaw j.
    mortise j. / ankle j.
    PIP / proximal interphalangeal j. / fingers and toes
    talocrural j. / ankle j.
Jones fracture / *of the fifth metatarsal*
J-point
JRA / juvenile rheumatoid arthritis
J-tubes
jugal / *connecting*
jugal bone / malar or zygomatic bone / *cheekbones*
jugular / *pertaining to the throat, neck or jugular vein*
jugular venous distention / JVD
jugular venous pressure / jugular venous pulse / JVP
junct / junction
justo major / justo minor (Ortho) / *pelvis area*
juxt / *near*
juxta-articular / *near a joint* / *in the region of a joint*
juxtallocortex (Neuro)
JVD / jugular venous distention

Additional Entries

____

____

____

____

K / *potassium*
kaleidoscope
kalemia / *potassium in blood*
Kanavel / *type of instrument*
Kaon-Cl / *potassium supplement* / D
Kaopectate / *antidiarrheal* / D
kappa
karyotype / *chromosome characteristic of cell*
katzenjammer / *hangover*
Kawasaki disease / *lymph node syndrome*
Kay Ciel / *potassium supplement* / D
Kayexalate / *potassium removing agent for hyperkalemia* / D
Kaye dissecting scissors
KCl / *potassium chloride*
K-Dur / *potassium supplement* / D
Keftab / *cephalosporin-type antibiotic* / D
Kefzol / cefazolin / *intramuscular or intravenous* / *surgical prophylaxis* / D
Kegel exercises (GU) / *for incontinence*
keloid / *scar*
Kenalog (Derm) / *topical corticosteroid* / D
Keralyte gel (discontinued 1994) / *topical keratolytic* / D
keratinous / *horny cyst*
keratitis (Oph) / *inflammation of the cornea*
keratoacanthoma / *benign epithelial tumor*
keratoconus (Oph) / *bilateral protrusion of the cornea*
keratoderma (Derm) / *a horny skin or covering*
keratosis / (pl.) keratoses / *horny growth*
keratosis, pilaris rubra / *hair follicles, thighs and arms*
keratotomy (Oph) / *incision of cornea*
Kerley-B lines / *chest x-ray*

Additional Entries

____

____

____

____

Kerlix
Kerlone / *antihypertensive* / D
Kernig sign / *sign of meningitis* / *leg extension*
keto- / *combining form for compounds containing a ketone*
ketoacidosis / *acidosis due to excess ketone bodies*
ketoconazole / *broad-spectrum antifungal* / D
ketone / *any of a class of organic compounds* / *k. acids are the end product of fat metabolism*
ketoprofen / *antiarthritic* / *nonsteroidal anti-inflammatory* / D
ketorolac tromethamine / Toradol / *analgesic* / *nonsteroidal anti-inflammatory drug* / D
ketotic (adj.), ketosis (n.) / *having elevated ketone bodies*
KG / kilogram
kidney, upper pole of
Kiesselbach area / *plexus*
Klaron / *for acne vulgaris* / D
K-Lease / *potassium supplement* / D
Klebsiella pneumoniae / *pulmonary infection* / *caused by Klebsiella bacteria*
Klonopin / clonazepam / *anticonvulsant* / D
Klor-Con / *potassium supplement* / D
Klorvess / *potassium supplement* / *effervescent tablets* / D
K-Lyte / *potassium supplement* / *effervescent tablets* / D
KOH / *potassium hydroxide* / D
koilocytotoxic / *infected with human papilloma virus of the uterus*
Kondremul / *laxative* / D
Konsyl / psyllium / *bulk laxative* / D [OTC]
Koplik spots / *on buccal and lingual mucosa*
Korotkoff sounds / *sounds heard during auscultatory determination of blood pressure*
K-Phos Neutral / *phosphorus supplement* / D

Additional Entries

____

____

____

____

K-Tab / potassium chloride / *potassium supplement* / D
KUB / kidney, ureters, bladder
Kussmaul breathing / *air hunger*
Kutapressen / *liver extract* / D
Ku-Zyme / *digestive enzymes* / D
Kwell / lindane / *cream* / *lotion* / *shampoo* / *for scabies,
    head lice, crab lice* / D
K-Y jelly / *vaginal lubricant*
kyphos / *a hump*
kyphoscoliosis (Ortho) / *lateral curvature of the spine with
    anteroposterior hump*
kyphosis (Ortho) / *bent spine* / *hunchback*
kyphotic (Ortho) / *affected by or pertaining to kyphosis*
Kytril / granisetron / *antiemetic* / *antinauseant* / *for chemo-
    therapy* / D

K

Additional Entries

L1—L5 / *first through fifth lumbar vertebrae or nerves*
lab / laboratory
labetalol / Normodyne / Trandate / *antiadrenergic* / D
labial abscess (Gyn)
labia majora, minora (Gyn)
labile / *unstable* / *unsteady* / *not fixed*
lability / *emotional*
labio- / *lips*
labrum / *liplike structure*
labyrinthine/-itis (Oto) / *internal ear*
Lacey LeBeau tea
Lachman exam (Ortho) / *knee*
Lac-Hydrin / *lotion* / *moisturizer* / *emollient* / D
lacerate / *to tear, as into irregular segments*
lacerability / *capability of being wounded or torn by a jagged instrument*
laceration / *a wound* / *an irregular tear of the flesh*
Lacri-Lube / *ocular moisturizer* / *lubricant* / D
LactAid / *for lactose intolerance*
LactiCare ointment / *emollient* / *moisturizer* / D [OTC]
Lactobacillus / *bacteria*
lactovegetarian / *eats only vegetables and dairy products, eschewing foods of animal origin*
lactovegan diet
Lactrase / *for lactose intolerance* / D
lactulose / *laxative*
lacunar infarct
LAD / left anterior descending
LAHB / LAH / left anterior hemiblock
lambliasis / giardiasis / *common infection of the small intestine*
Lamictal / *anti-epileptic* / D

Additional Entries

____

____

____

____

lamina propria / *tympanic or mucous membrane*
laminectomy / *excision of the posterior arch of a vertebra*
Lamisil / *systemic antifungal for onychomycosis* / D
Lamprene / *bactericidal* / *tuberculostatic* / *leprostatic* / D
Lanacaine / benzocaine / *topical local anesthetic* / D
Lanacort / hydrocortisone / *topical corticosteroid* / D
lancets / *needles* / *diabetes test* / T
lancinating / *sharp pain*
Lanoxicaps / digoxin / *cardiac glycoside* / *antiarrhythmic* / D
Lanoxin / digoxin / *cardiac glycoside* / *antiarrhythmic* / D
laparo- / *the loins*
laparoscopy / *abdominal exploration using a laparoscope*
laparotomy / *surgical opening of the abdomen*
Lariam / mefloquine / *for malaria* / D
laryn-, laryngo- / *the larynx* / *voice box*
laryngeal / *pertaining to the larynx*
laryngopharyngitis / *inflammation of the larynx and the pharynx*
laryngotracheal / *pertaining to the larynx and the trachea*
larynx / *voice box*
Lasegue / *straight leg*
Lasix / furosemide / *loop diuretic* / D
L-asparaginase / D
late potential (Cardio)
latissimus / *a muscle in upper torso*
LAV / lymphadenopathy-associated virus
lavage / *washing*
laxity / *looseness* / *lacking firmness*
LBBB (Cardio) / left bundle branch block
LD / lethal dose
LDH elevation / lactic dehydrogenase (elevation)
LDL / low density lipoprotein / *the "bad cholesterol"*

Additional Entries

____

____

____

____

12-lead electrocardiogram
Ledercillin / *bactericidal antibiotic* / D
LEEP (Gyn) / loop electrosurgical excision procedure
Legg-Calvé-Perthes disease / *osteochondritis*
Legionella / *bacteria* / *from Philadelphia 1976 Legionnaire disease*
leio- / *smooth*
leiomyoma / *tumor of mostly smooth muscle tissue*
leiomyosarcoma (Onc) / *combined leiomyoma and sarcoma*
lens opacities, bilaterally (Oph)
Lente / *pork insulin* / *for diabetes* / D
lentigo / (pl.) lentigines (Derm) / *melanosis on the skin*
-lepsis, -lepsy / *seizure* / e.g., epi**lepsy**
lepto- / *frail* / *light* / *thin*
leptodactylous / *thin fingers*
leptodermic / *thin skin*
Lescol / *cholesterol-lowering antihyperlipidemic* / D
Letterer-Siwe disease / *early childhood disease characterized by eczema, enlarged liver and spleen, and anemia*
leucovorin / Wellcovorin / *chemotherapy "rescue"* / D
leuk- / *white* / *color*
Leukeran / chlorambucil / *antineoplastic* / D
leukemoid reaction
leukocytoclastic
leukocytosis / *increase in number of leukocytes*
leukopenia / *abnormal decrease in white blood cells*
leukoplakia / *on mucous membrane, white patch that will not rub off*
levamisole / *antineoplastic* / D
Levatol / *antihypertensive* / *beta blocker* / D
LeVeen Shunt / *tube used to transport ascitic fluid from abdomen*
Levlen 28 / *oral contraceptive* / D

L

Additional Entries

levodopa / *for Parkinson disease* / D
levoscoliosis / *S-shaped spine*
Levothroid / levothyroxine / *thyroid hormone* / D
Levoxyl / levothyroxine / *thyroid hormone* / D
Levoxine (named changed to Levoxyl in 1994) / D
Levsin / *sedative* / D
Levsinex Timecaps / *antispasmodic* / D
LFS / liver function series
LFTs / liver function test / T
LH / luteinizing hormone / T
Lhemitte sign / *disorder of cervical cord* / *when person bends head,*
    electric shocks go down body
Librax / *anxiolytic* / D
Librium / *anxiolytic* / D
lichen chronicus simplex (Derm) / *eczematous dermatitis*
lichen sclerosus et atrophicus (Derm)
lichenification (Derm) / *leathery skin*
lichen planus / *fungus* / (pronounced "lye-ken")
Lidex-E / *cream* / *relief of pain*
lidocaine-1% / *5ml vial viscous* / *topical local anesthetic* / D
Life Stream / *self-help group*
lifts / heaves (Cardio)
ligamentous tear
Ligamentum flavum
Limbitrol / amitriptyline / *antidepressant* / *anxiolytic* / D
Lincocin / lincomycin / *antibiotic* / D
lindane 1% cream / *pediculicide* / *scabicide* / D
linea semilunaris / *rectus muscle*
lingua / *tongue* / *structure*
    (also related) **gloss-** / *disease* / *injury* / *to tongue*
lingula / *a small tonguelike structure*

Additional Entries

____

____

____

____

liniment cream
Lioresal / *skeletal muscle relaxant* / D
lip- / *fat* / *fatty tissue*
lipedema / *accumulation of fat in subcutaneous tissues*
lipid-lowering medication
lipid profile / *lab test* / T
Lipisorb / *enteral nutritional therapy* / D
Lipitor-HMG-CoA / *reductase inhibitor* / D
lipoflavonoid
lipogranuloma / *inflammation and granulation of fatty tissue*
lipoma/-s / *fatty tumor*
lipomatosis / *excessive deposit of fat in localized area*
liponephrosis
lipoprotein
liquefaction / *conversion of a material into liquid form*
Liquibid / *expectorant* / D
Lisfranc joint / *between foot and leg*
lisinopril / *antihypertensive* / *ACE inhibitor for congestive heart
    failure and myocardial infarction* / D
Lispro / *drug study*
lith- / *stone* / *abnormal formation* / e.g., **lith**iasis
lithium / *element* / D
Lithobid / *antipsychotic* / D
lithotomy / *cutting operation for removal of calculus*
lithotripsy / *crushing of calculus with mechanical force or
    sound waves*
livedo reticularis / *discolored skin*
liver enzyme elevation
livid / *black and blue or gray color*
lobo- / *section* / *well-defined (lobe) of brain, glands, or organs*
lobectomy / *surgical removal of a lobe of an organ or gland*

L

Additional Entries

lobular / *lobe-shaped* / *pertaining to a lobe*
Locoid cream / topical corticosteroid / D
loculated pus
loculus / *cavity*
locum tenens / *one serving in a temporary office or capacity*
Lodine / etodolac / *analgesic* / *for arthritis pain* / D
Lodosyn / carbidopa / *for Parkinson Disease* / D
Loestrin Fe / *oral contraceptive* / *iron supplement* / D
lomefloxacin / Maxaquin / *antibacterial* / D
Lomotil / *for diarrhea* / D
lone episode / *only happened once*
longissimus dorsi / *long muscles, posterior*
long-/short-leg / *splint or cast*
long tract signs
Loniten / minoxidil / *antihypertensive* / *vasodilator* / D
loop diuretics
loopogram
loose bodies
Lo-Ovral / *contraceptive* / D
Lopid / gemfibrozil / *antihyperlipidemic agent* / D
Lopidine / D
Lopressor / metoprolol tartrate / *antihypertensive* / D
Loprox cream / *topical antifungal* / D
Lorabid / loracarbef / *antibiotic* / D
lorazepam / Ativan / *anxiolytic* / *minor tranquilizer* / D
Lorcet Plus / hydrocodone and acetaminophen / *narcotic analgesic*/D
lordosis/-otic / *deformity* / *curvature of spine*
Lorelco / *for serum cholesterol reduction* / D
Lortab / hydrocodone and acetaminophen / *narcotic analgesic*/ D
losartan / Cozaar / D
Losec / omeprazole / *foreign name for Prilosec* / D

Additional Entries

____
____
____
____

Lotensin / HCT / benazepril hydrochloride / *antihypertensive* / D

Lotrel 5/10 / amlodipine and benazepril / *antihypertensive* / D

Lotrimin solution / *topical antifungal* / D [OTC]

Lotrisone / betamethasone and clotrimazole / *topical corticosteroid* / *antifungal* / D

lovastatin / Mevacor / *antihypercholesterolemic* / D

Low-Dye / *strap*

Loxitane / loxapine / *antipsychotic* / D

Lozol / *antihypertensive* / *diuretic* / D

LP / lumbar puncture

LSO / left salpingo-oophorectomy

lucency/-ies / *punctate* / *points or dots*

Ludiomil / maprotiline / *tetracyclic antidepressant* / D

lues / *a plague* / *syphilis*

Lufyllin / dyphylline / *bronchodilator* / D

lumbar / *pertaining to the loin or loins* / *the part of the back between the thorax and the pelvis* / e.g., l. vertebra; l. artery

lumbar lordosis / *hollow back* / *swayback* / *saddleback*

lumbosacral / *pertaining to the lumbar vertebrae and the sacrum*

lumbosyringomyelia

lunula/-ae / *nail*

lunate bone / *moon-shaped*

lung fields

Lupron / *hormonal chemotherapy for prostate cancer* / D

lupus erythematosus / *connective tissue disorder*

luteal / *pertaining to corpus luteum, its cells, or its hormone*

luteinize/-ing / *forming luteal tissue*

luteum (Gyn) / *yellow cellular mass formed in the ovary*

Luvox / *antidepressant* / D

Additional Entries

LVH / left ventricular hypertrophy
Lyme disease / *characterized by arthritis and myalgia*
Lyme titer / *lab*
lymphadenitic / *streaking*
lymphadenopathy / *disease of lymph nodes*
lymphangitis/-itic / *inflammation of lymphatic channels or vessels*
lymphedema praecox / *swelling of lower limbs in females at or
    near puberty*
lymphedema pump / *for draining excess body fluid*
lymphocytic/-osis
lymphogranuloma venereum / *an infectious venereal disease*
lymphoproliferative / *pertaining to proliferation of lymphoid tissue*
lyo- / *loosen* / *dissolve*
lyomyoma
lyomyosarcoma
lyse/-es / *lyze* / *break up* / *disintegrate*
lysis / *gradual decrease of disease symptoms*
-lysis / *free* / *loosen* / *dissolve* / *decompose* / *destruct*
lytes / *electrolytes*
lytic / *pertaining to lysis* / *colloquial abbreviation for "osteolytic"*

Additional Entries

____

____

____

____

macerate/-ation / *soften by wetting*
Machida scope
macr-, **macro-** / *large* / *long* / e.g., **macro**podia
Macrobid / *urinary bacteriostatic* / D
macrobiota / *the combined plants and animals of a region*
macrobiote / *an organism that is long-lived*
macrobiotic / *tending to prolong life*
macrobiotic diet / *promoting well-being and longevity by eating a diet of whole grains and beans*
macrobiotics / *the study of prolongation of life*
macrocytic anemia / *abnormally large erythrocytes*
macrocytosis
Macrodantin / *urinary bacteriostatic* / D
macroglobulinemia / *increase in macroglobulins in the blood*
macropodia / megalopodia / *abnormally large feet*
macula (Oph) / *scar of the cornea*
maculopapular / *eruption consisting of both macules and papules*
Mag-Ox 400 / *antacid* / *magnesium supplement* / D [OTC]
Maisonneuve (Ortho) / *fracture of fibula*
majora / minora, labia
-malacia / *morbid softening of a part or tissue*
malaise / *bodily discomfort and fatigue*
malar / *cheek* / *cheek bones*
Malassezia furfur (Derm) / *type of fungus normal on human skin, that causes tinea versicolor in susceptible individuals*
malathion / Ovide / *for head lice and their ova* / D
malingering / *feigning illness or disability*
mallei / malleus (Oto) / *an auditory ossicle in the middle ear*
malleolus/-i/-ar (Ortho) / *a rounded process, as either side of ankle joint*
Mallinckrodt

Additional Entries

____

____

____

____

Mallory-Weiss syndrome / *hematemesis or melena following hours or days of severe vomiting*
Maltese cross
mammilate/-ed / *covered with nipplelike projections*
mammillation / *the breast / nipplelike projection*
mammoplasty (Gyn) / *plastic reconstruction of the breast*
Mandelamine / *urinary bactericidal* / D
mandible/-ular / *the bones of the lower jaw* / e.g., m. angle
maneuvers, Nylen and Bárány (Oto) / *test for benign positional vertigo* / T
mani- / *madness / loss of control over emotions / nerves / mental processes*
manometry / *measure of pressure of liquids or gases*
mantle / *covering layer*
manubrium / (pl.) -ia (Ortho) / *part of the sternum*
maprotiline / Ludiomil / *for depression* / D
Marcaine / bupivacaine / *injectable local anesthetic* / D
march fracture / *fracture of foot due to continued trauma with repetitive activity* / e.g., injury to feet of marching soldiers
march hematuria / *hematuria secondary to trauma of repetitive activity* / e.g., in marching soldiers, impact breaks up red cells, which are excreted in the urine
marfanoid body habitus / *abnormal length of the extremities*
marijuana / cannabis / hashish
markedly tender
Marshall-Marchetti / *operation* / T
Marlex mesh / *synthetic graft material / for tissue reinforcement*
masseter / *muscle*
mast-, masto- / *breast / front of chest* / e.g., **mast**ectomy
    also... *pertaining to chewing* / e.g., **mast**oid, **mast**ication
mastocytosis

Additional Entries

____

____

____

____

mastodynia / *breast pain*
mastoiditis / *inflammation* / *infection of mastoid air cells*
MAT / multifocal atrial tachycardia
matricectomy / *removal of uterus*
matrix / (pl.) -ices / *tissue from which a structure develops*
Mavik / trandolapril / *antihypertensive* / D
Maxair Inhaler / *bronchodilator for bronchospasm* / D
Maxaquin / lomefloxacin hydrochloride / *broad-spectrum antibiotic* / D
Maxivate / betamethasone / *lotion* / *topical corticosteroid* / D
Maxzide / hydrochlorothiazide / *antihypertensive* / *diuretic* / D
McBurney point / *incision*

M

mcg / *microgram*
MCHC / Mean Corpuscular Hemoglobin Concentration / L
McMurray test / M. sign (Ortho) / *manipulation of tibia with leg flexed produces distinct click if meniscus has been injured*
MCP joints / metacarpophalangeal (joints)
MCV, MCH / Mean Corpuscular Volume, Mean Corpuscular Hemoglobin / L.
MD / muscular dystrophy
MDI / multidose inhaler
M/E ratio / myeloid-erythroid (ratio)
meatus / meatal / *an opening or passageway in the body*
Mebaral / mephobarbital / *sedative* / *hypnotic* / *anticonvulsive* / D
mebendazole / *anthelmintic* / *treatment for worms* / D
Meckel diverticulum / *appendage of the ileum*
meclizine / *for vertigo* / *antiemetic* / *antihistamine* / D
Meclomen (discontinued 1996) / *nonsteroidal anti-inflammatory* / D
MEDCO Sonicator
medial components / *pertaining to the middle*

Additional Entries

medialis / *structure situated nearer to the midline of a body*

mediastinum/-al/-oscopy / *tissues and organs separating the two pleural sacs*

mediated / *accomplished by the aid of an intervening medium*

medicamentosus / *overmedicated*

medium inspiratory / *rales* / *sounds of fluid in the lungs*

Medjugorje

medullary / medullar / *pertaining to marrow or medulla* / *resembling marrow*

Medrol Dosepak / methylprednisolone / *glucocorticoid* / *anti-inflammatory* / D

medroxyprogesterone / *progestin* / *antineoplastic* / D

meds / medications

Mefoxin / cefoxitin / *injection* / *antibiotic* / D

Megace / megestrol acetate / *antineoplastic* / *for breast or endometrial cancer* / D

megakaryocytes/-cytic / *the giant cell of bone marrow*

megal-, -megalo-, megaly- / *enlarged* / *abnormal increase in size* / e.g., **megalo**blastoid, hepato**megaly**

megaloblastoid/-tic / *immature progenitor of an abnormal red blood cell*

megalopodia / macropodia / *abnormally large feet*

meibomianitis (Oph) / *inflammation of the meibomian gland*

meiosis / *cell division*

melan- / *black* / *color*

melanosis coli / *mucous membrane of colon is dark brown due to pigment within*

melanotic / *having the presence of melanin*

melasma / *blotchy* / *brown facial discoloration* / *"mask of pregnancy"*

melena / *black stool*

Additional Entries

---

melatonin / *sleep aid* / D

Mellaril / thioridazine / *antipsychotic* / D

meloplasty / *plastic surgery of the cheek*

Memorial Sloan-Kettering Hospital, NY

MEN / multiple endocrine neoplasia/neoplasms

menarche / menarchal / *beginning menses*

Ménétrier disease (GI) / *giant hypertrophic gastritis*

Meniere disease / M. syndrome / *characterized by hearing loss, tinnitus, sensation of pressure in ears, and vertigo*

mening-, meningo- / *the meninges* / *the three membranes that envelop the brain and spinal cord*

meningeal / *pertaining to the meninges*

meninges (plural of meninx) / *membranes, especially of the brain and spinal cord*

meningioma / *vascular tumor*

meningismus / meningism / *irritation of brain and spinal cord in which symptoms simulate meningitis, but without actual inflammation*

meningitis / Listeria / *bacterial or viral inflammation of meninges*
meningococcal

meningomyelocele / *hernia of spinal cord and membranes*

meninx / (pl.) meninges / *membrane covering brain or spinal cord*

meniscal (Ortho) / *dome-shaped cartilage*

meniscal tearing (Ortho) / *tearing of meniscus cartilage of knee*

meniscectomy (Ortho) / *removal of meniscus cartilage of knee*

meniscus/-ci (Ortho) / *knee cartilage*

meno- / *menses* / *menstruation*

menorrhagia (Gyn) / hypermenorrhea / *excessive uterine bleeding during menses*

menometrorrhagia (Gyn) / *excessive uterine bleeding both during menses and at other intervals*

Additional Entries

Menrium / *estrogen replacement therapy* / *for postmenopausal disorders* / D
menses (Gyn) / *monthly flow of bloody fluid from uterus*
mentation / *mental activity*
Mepergan Fortis / *analgesic* / *sedative* / D
meperidine / *narcotic analgesic* / D
Mephyton / phytonadione / *coagulant* / D
meprazole...**NO!** (see "Omeprazole") / D
meprobamate / *anxiolytic* / D
mEq / *milliequivalents*
meralgia paresthetica / *burning, prickling, numbness or pain in the thigh*
6-mercaptopurine / 6-MP / *antimetabolic antineoplastic* / D
Mercurochrome / *antiseptic* / D
mere-, mero- / *part* / *one of a series of similar parts*
meromicrosomia / *abnormal smallness of body part* / *local dwarfism*
merosmia / *inability to smell certain odors*
merthiolate (discontinued 1992) / *antiseptic* / *antifungal* / D
mesalamine / Pentasa Oral / *anti-inflammatory* / *for ulcerative colitis* / D
mesangial proliferation (Uro)
mesangiopathic (Uro)
mesenteric artery syndrome, superior
mesentery / *portion of peritoneum attached to abdominal wall and enclosing certain vessels and nerves*
mesna / Mesnex injection / *urotoxic antidote* / *for urotoxicity* / D
mesothelial / *flat cells lining the body cavity of the embryo*
mesothelioma / *tumor of peritoneum, pleura or pericardium*
mesothelium/-ia / *cells forming an epithelium that lines serous cavities* / *e.g., pleura; pericardium*
Mestinon / pyridostigmine bromide / *muscle stimulant* / D

Additional Entries

metacarpal (Ortho) / *the part of the hand between the wrist and the fingers*

Metamucil / psyllium / *bulk laxative* / D

metamyelocyte / *transitional form of a type of young cell (myelocyte) found in bone marrow*

metanephrine / *metabolite of epinephrine excreted in urine*

metaphysics

metaphysis (Ortho) / *part of a long bone that contains the growth zone*

metaplasia / *change of normal cells in a tissue to abnormal cells for that tissue*

Metaprel inhaler / *bronchodilator* / D

metastasis / metastatic / *transfer of disease from one organ to another*

metastasize / *spread of disease from one part of the body to another*

metatarsal (Ortho) / *pertaining to metatarsus or metatarsal bones*

metatarsalgia (Ortho) / *pain in fore part of the foot*

metatarsophalangeal (Ortho)

metathesis / *the artificial transfer of a morbid process*

meters squared / m^2

metformin / Glucophage / *antidiabetic* / D

methacholine / *cholinergic* / D

methadone / *narcotic analgesic* / D

methicillin resistant staph aureus / MRSA / *in pneumonia*

methiolate...**NO!** (see "merthiolate")

methocarbamol / *skeletal muscle relaxant* / D

methotrexate / amethopterin / mtx / *antineoplastic* / *for leukemia, psoriasis, rheumatoid arthritis* / D

methyldopa / *antihypertensive* / D

methylmalonic acid

Additional Entries

methylphenidate / Ritalin / *central nervous system (CNS) stimulant for attention deficit hyperactivity disorders (ADHD)* / D
methylprednisolone / *anti-inflammatory* / *immunosuppressant* / D
Metimyd / (Oph) / *eye drops* / *topical corticosteroid* / D
metoclopramide / *antiemetic for chemotherapy* / D
MET I program
metoprolol / Lopressor / Toprol / *antihypertensive* / D
MetroGel Topical / metronidazole / *for acne rosacea* / D
metronidazole / MetroGel Topical / *antibiotic* / *amebicide* / D
metrorrhagia (Gyn) / *completely irregular but frequent uterine bleeding*
Mevacor / lovastatin / *cholesterol-lowering antihyperlipidemic* / D
Mexitil / mexiletine / *antiarrhythmic* / D
MF heel cup
mg / milligram
mg/dl / milligrams per deciliter
MI (Cardio) / myocardial infarction
Miacalcin nasal spray / *calcium regulator for postmenopausal osteoporosis* / D
Micatin / *foot powder* / *anti-fungal* / D [OTC]
Mi-Cebrin-T / *vitamin/mineral/iron supplement* / D [OTC]
miconazole / *antifungal agent* / D
micr-, micro- / *small*
microadenoma / *small adenoma in pituitary*
Micro-K / potassium chloride / D
microalbuminuria
microaneurysm / *microscopic retinal aneurysm characteristic of diabetes mellitus*
microbacterium / *small, rod-shaped bacteria found in dairy products*
microcalcifications / *tiny calcifications* / *in breast*
microcardia / *abnormally small heart*

Additional Entries

---

microcytic red cells / *abnormally small erythrocytes*
microcytosis / *many microcytes in circulating blood*
micrognathia / *small jaw*
microhematuria / *small blood cells in the urine*
micrometastasis (Gyn) / *state of metastasis with tumors too small to be clinically detected*
micromyelia / *abnormally small or short spinal cord*
Micronase / glyburide / *sulfonylurea antidiabetic* / D
Micronor / norethindrone / *oral contraceptive* / D
Microspacer
micturate / micturition / *urinate*
MID / multi-infarct dementia
Midamor / amiloride hydrochloride / *potassium-sparing diuretic* / D
mid-bulb
midline
mid lumbar region
Midrin / acetaminophen / *sedative analgesic* / D
midsystolic
migraine / migrainous / *periodic attacks of vascular headaches*
milestones
milia / *whitehead*
miliaria rubra
milium / *cyst*
milk of bismuth / *used as an astringent* / antacid
millimoles / mmol
min / *minute*
mineralocorticoid
Minimental / *test for forgetfulness* / T
Minipress / prazosin / *antihypertensive* / D
Minitran patch / *nitroglycerin* / D

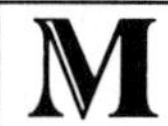

Additional Entries

____

____

____

____

Minocin / minocycline hydrochloride / *treatment of acne and
bacterial infections* / D
minocycline hydrochloride / Minocin / D
minoxidil / Loniten / Minodyl / Rogaine / *hair growth stimulant* / D
Mintezol / thiabendazole / *anthelmintic* / *destructive to worms* / D
miosis / myosis
miotic / myotic
mirabile dictu / *"wonderful to relate"*
mirabilis, Proteus
misoprostol / Cytotec / *prevention of nonsteroidal anti-inflammatory drug (NSAID)-induced gastic ulcers* / D
mithramycin / *antibiotic antineoplastic* / D
mitomycin / Mutamycin / D
mitotic / *pertaining to cell reproduction* / *indirect division of a cell*
Mito-Velban / D
mitoxantrone HCl / Novantrone / *antibiotic antineoplastic* / D
mitral commisurotomy (Cardio) / *surgical procedure to increase
size of mitral valve orifice* / *used in treating mitral stenosis*
mitral stenosis (Cardio) / *constriction or narrowing of mitral valve
or orifice of heart, or both*
mitral valve prolapse / MVP / (Cardio)
mittelschmerz / *intermenstrual pain* / *ovulation pain*
ml / milliliter
ml/min / milliliters per minute
ml/sec / milliliters per second
mm / millimeter
mmHg / millimeters of mercury
mmol / millimoles
mmol/l / millimoles per liter
MMR / measles, mumps, rubella / *vaccine*
Moban (Psych) / molindone hydrochloride / D

Additional Entries

Mobitz (Cardio) / *heart block*
Mobius syndrome / *inability to keep the eyes converged* /
    in Graves disease
moccasin
Modane / *laxative* / D [OTC]
Modicon / *oral contraceptive* / D
modicum / *small amount*
Moduretic / *diuretic* / *antihypertensive* / D
Moh / *scale* / *technique* / *surgery*
molimen / (pl.) -a / *great effort to perform normal function*
molimina of puffiness / *unpleasant symptom preceding the*
    mentrual period
Mollaret meningitis
molluscum contagiosum (Derm) / *contagious skin disease*
MOM / Milk of Magnesia / *antacid* / *electrolyte supplement* /
    laxative / D [OTC]
Momentum / *anti-inflammatory* / *analgesic* / D
mon-, mono- / *alone* / *single* / *one* / *one part*
monarticular / monoarticular / *a single joint*
Monilia / Candida / *monilial vaginitis*
moniliasis / candidiasis / *yeastlike fungi*
Monistat Dual-Pak / miconazole / *cream* / *vaginal suppositories* /D
mono / *colloquial term for mononucleosis*
monoblastic leukemia
Monocid / cefonicid sodium / *antibiotic for injection* / D
monoclonal / *a protein from a single clone of cells*
mononucleosis / *abnormally large number of mononuclear leuko-*
    cytes in the blood / also ... infectious m.
monoparesis / *partial or incomplete paralysis of one limb*
monoplegia / *paralysis of one limb*
Monopril / fosinopril / *antihypertensive* / D

Additional Entries

Monospot / *diagnostic aid for mononucleosis* / T
mons pubis (Gyn) / *the prominent fatty pad over the symphysis pubis*
Monteggia (Ortho) / *arm fracture*
morbilliform / *resembling measles rash* / *like measles*
Morganella morganii / *type of bacteria*
Moro / *reflex Peds*
morph-, morpho- / form / shape / structure
morpheaform basal cell / *localized form of scleroderma*
morphologically / *pertaining to the form and structure of an organism, organ or part*
mortise (Ortho)
motor radiculopathy
motor strength 5+ out of 5+ (Neuro)
MRI / magnetic resonance imaging / *scan*
MRSA / methicillin-resistant staph aureus
MS Contin / morphine sulfate (Contin) / D
MSEL / myasthenic syndrome of Eaton-Lambert
M spike / monoclonal s. / *abnormal accumulation of proteins in one area on protein electrophoresis*
MTP joints / metatarsophalangeal (joints)
mucocele / *type of cyst*
mucoepidermoid / *carcinoma* / *salivary glands*
mucoid / *resembling mucus*
mucoperichondrial flaps
mucoperiosteal / *consisting of mucous membrane and periosteum*
mucopurulent / *mucous discharge containing pus*
mucosal
mucous (*adj.*) / *relating to a mucus or a m. membrane*
mucous membrane
mucus (*noun*) / *secretion of the mucous membranes*

Additional • Entries

____

____

____

____

MUGA / multigated angiogram / *exercise treadmill test*

Muenster cast

multiagent chemotherapy

multifactorial / *arising through the action of many factors*

multinodular goiter

multiphasic

mupirocin / *topical antibacterial antibiotic* / D

mural / *pertaining to the wall of any body cavity*

mural thrombus (Cardio)

murmur (II/VI) (Cardio)

Murphy's sign

muscularis / *the muscular covering of a hollow organ or tubular structure*

musculoskeletal / *pertaining to both muscles and skeleton*

Muse therapy / *for erectile dysfunction*

Mustargen / mechlorethamine / *antineoplastic* / *for multiple myelomas and breast, lung and ovarian cancers* / D

MVA / motor vehicle accident

M-VAC (Chemo) / D

MVI / multivitamins

MVV (Pulm) / maximum voluntary ventilation

my- / *muscle* / e.g., **my**algia / *muscle pain*

Myadec / *vitamin* / *mineral/iron supplement* / D

Myambutol / ethambutol / *tuberculostatic* / D

myasthenia gravis / *disorder of neuromuscular function* / *of eye, face, lips, tongue, throat and neck*

myatonia / *deficiency or loss of muscular tone*

Mycelex / clotrimazole / *cream* / *antifungal* / D

Mycelex troches / *for oral candidiasis* / D

mycet-, myceto-, myco / *fungus* / e.g., **mycet**oma, **myco**stat

mycetes / *fungi*

Additional Entries

---

mycetoma / *progressive, destructive infection caused by aerobic actinomycetes or fungi*
Mycitracin / bacitracin / *topical antibiotic* / D
myco-, mycet-, myceto- / *fungus*
Mycobacterium avium intracellulare / *organisms that cause human pulmonary disease and lymphadenitis in children*
Mycobacterium kansasii / *etiologic agent of a tuberculosislike disease in humans*
Mycobacterium marinum / *found in aquariums, diseased fish, and swimming pools*
Mycocide NS / *nail solution* / *topical antiseptic* / D [OTC]
Mycolog-II / *topical corticosteroid* / D
Mycolog / *cream* / *topical corticosteroid* / *antifungal* / D
Mycoplasma / *parasites and pathogens distributed on the mucous membranes of humans, animals and birds*
mycoplasmal pneumonia
mycosis/-es/-cotic / *any disease caused by a fungus*
mycosis fungoides / *cutaneous T-cell lymphoma*
mycostasis / *stopping the growth of fungi*
mycostat / *anything that stops the growth of fungi*
Mycostatin elixir / *antifungal* / D
myelin/-ic / *soft, white, fatty substance encasing the axis cylinder of certain nerve fibers*
myelinization
myelodysplasia / *abnormal spinal cord, especially lower part*
myelodysplastic /
myelofibrosis / *fibrosis of bone marrow*
myelogenous leukemia
myelogram
myeloid basic protein
myeloma / *tumor composed of certain bone marrow cells*

Additional Entries

---

myelopathy / *spinal cord disorder*
myeloproliferative / *abnormal growth of bone marrow tissue*
Mykrox / metolazone / *diuretic / antihypertensive* / D
Myleran / busulfan / *antineoplastic / for myelogenous leukemia* / D
Mylicon / simethicone / *antiflatulent* / D
myocardial infarction / MI (Cardio)
myocardium (Cardio) / *muscle of the heart*
myoclonic / *muscle*
myoclonus
myofascial / *pertaining to fascia surrounding and separating muscle tissue*
Myoflex / *cream / topical analgesic* / D
myoglobinuria / *presence of myoglobin in urine*
myoma / *benign tumor consisting of muscle tissue*
myomectomy / *surgical removal of a myoma, specifically a uterine myoma*
myometrial (Gyn) / *pertaining to the myometrium, muscular wall of the uterus*
myopalmus / *twitching of muscles*
myopathy / *any disease or abnormal condition of striated muscle*
myositis ossificans / *bone in muscle, resulting in pain and swelling*
myotonic dystrophy / *progressive disease characterized by muscle weakness and wasting*
myring-, myringo- / *eardrum*
myringa (Oto) / *the tympanic membrane*
myringitis (Oto) / *inflammation of the tympanum or eardrum*
myringomycosis (Oto) / *inflammation of the tympanic membrane from infection by parasitic fungi*
Mysoline / primidone / *anticonvulsant* / D
Mytrex cream / *topical / corticosteroid / antifungal* / D

Additional Entries

---

myx-, myxo- / mucus
myxedema/-atous / *hypothyroidism characterized by severe edema*
myxoma nabothian (Gyn) / *cyst*

Additional Entries

nabothian cyst (Gyn) / *retention cyst formed when a mucous gland of the cervix uteri is obstructed*
nabumetone / Relafen / *nonsteroidal anti-inflammatory / for arthritis* / D
NAD / no appreciable disease
nadir / *the lowest possible point* / (opposite) *zenith*
nadolol / *antianginal / antihypertensive* / D
nafarelin / Synarel / *hormone-releasing hormone agonist* / D
nafcillin / *antibacterial* / D
Naldecon / *decongestant / antihistamine* / D
Naldecon Senior / EX / *liquid expectorant* / D
Nalfon / *nonsteroidal anti-inflammatory* / D
NANB / non-A, non-B (hepatitis)
Naphcon-A (Oph) / *eye drops / topical ocular decongestant* / D
Naprelan / naproxen / *nonsteroidal anti-inflammatory* / D
Naprosyn / naproxen / *nonsteroidal anti-inflammatory* / D
naproxen / Aleve (OTC) / Anaprox / Naprosyn / *analgesic / antiarthritic* / D
Naqua / trichlormethiazide / *diuretic / antihypertensive* / D
Narcan / naloxone / *narcotic antagonist / for opiate dependence* / D
Nardil / phenelzine / *antidepressant / antipsychotic* / D
nares / *nostrils*
Nasacort / triamcinolone / *nasal spray / intranasal steroidal anti-inflammatory* / D
Nasalcrom / *nasal spray / bronchodilator / for bronchial asthma* / D
Nasalide / *nasal spray / intranasal steroidal anti-inflammatory* / D
nasal septoplasty / *surgical correction of nasal septum deformities*
nasal turbinates / *bones in the nose*
Nasarel inhaler / *intranasal steroidal anti-inflammatory* / D
nasogastric / *pertaining to the nose and stomach*
nasolabial folds / *pertaining to the nose and upper lip*

Additional Entries

____

____

____

____

nauseate

Navane (Psych) / *antipsychotic* / D

navicula/-ar / scaphoid / *small, boat-shaped structure*

NCT / number connection tests

NDC / nondifferentiated cells

neck, no JVD / *(neck, no) jugular venous distention*

necro-, nec- / *death* / e.g., **necro**sis

necrobiosis / *cell or tissue death*

necrobiosis lipoidica / *development of shiny yellow lesions on legs /*
 often associated with diabetes

necrocytosis / *process that results in abnormal or pathological*
 death of cells

necrosis / necrotic / *cell death*

nedocromil sodium / Tilade / *prophylactic antiallergic / anti-*
 asthmatic / D

neg / *negative*

NegGram / *urinary bactericidal* / D

Neisseria, gonorrhea / *bacteria species that causes gonorrhea and*
 other infections

Neisseria, meningitides (pl.) / *bacteria species found in nasopharynx*
 that causes meningococcal meningitis

Nélaton's catheter

Nembutal / *sedative / hypnotic* / D

nemonic...**NO!** / (see "mnemonic")

Neo-Calglucon / *calcium supplement* / D [OTC]

NeoDecadron ointment / *topical corticosteroid* / D

neo- / *new / recent*

neonatal / *pertaining to the period immediately after birth and*
 continuing for 28 days

neonatal placing

neonatology

Additional Entries

---

neoplasia / neoplasm / *abnormal new tissue growth*
Neoprene brace
Neosporin / *topical antibiotic* / D [OTC]
Neo-Synephrine / *nasal decongestant* / D
NEPD / no evidence of pulmonary disease
nephrectomy / *surgical removal of kidney*
nephro-, nephr- / *kidney* / *kidneys*
nephrolithiasis / *condition in which renal calculi are present*
nephropathy / *any kidney disease*
nephropexy (Uro) / *surgical fixation of a floating kidney*
nephrosclerosis
nephrostolithotomy / *removal of renal stone through nephrostomy tube, through abdominal wall into renal pelvis*
nephrotic
nephrotomogram / *sectional radiograph of the kidney*
nephroureterectomy / *excision of a kidney and part of the ureter*
Neptazane / methazolamide (Oph) / *carbonic anhydrase inhibitor* / *diuretic* / *for glaucoma* / D
nerve conductions
neur-, neuri-, neuro- / *nerve* / *nerve tissue* / *nervous system*
neural / *neurological*
neural foramina / *natural opening or passage into or through a bone, for the passage of nerves or blood vessels*
neuralgia / *nerve pain*
neurapraxia/-is / *least severe form of focal nerve lesion that causes clinical deficits*
neurectomy
neurinoma
neuro: cranial nerves II-XII
Neurocysticercosis

Additional Entries

____
____
____
____

neurocyte / neuron
neurodermatitis / *chronic skin lesion*
neuroectodermal / *portion of the ectoderm that gives rise to the central nervous system* (CNS)
neurofibromatosis
neuroforaminal
neurogenic/-ous / *pertaining to nervous tissue or impulses* / e.g., n. atrophy
neuro-imaging
neuro / neurology
neuroma, Morton's / *of the hand*
neuronitis / *inflammation of one or more neurons*
Neurontin / gabapentin / *anticonvulsant* / D
neuropathy / *any disease of the nerves*
neuropraxia...**NO!** (see "neur**a**praxia")
neuroroentgenography
neuro-urologic
neurovascular sheath
Neutra-Phos (discontinued 1994) / *phosphorus supplement* / D
Neutrogena / *topical cleanser for acne*
neutropenia
neutrophils
nevi / plural of nevus (Derm) / *skin disorder*
nevus / (pl.) nevi (Derm)
ng / nanogram
ng/ml / nanograms per milliliter
niacin / *vitamin B$_3$* / *vasodilator* / *antihyperlipidemic* / D
nicardipene / Cardene (Cardio) / *vasodilator* / *calcium channel blocker* / D
nicking (Oph) / *retinal*
Nicobid / *niacin therapy* / D

Additional Entries

____

____

____

____

Nicoderm patch / *smoking deterrent / nicotine withdrawal aid* / D

Nicotinex / *elixir / vitamin supplement* / D [OTC]

nidus / *point of origin*

nifedipine / *coronary vasodilator* / D

Niferex / *hematinic* / D

Nike shoe

Nissen fundoplication / *fundic wrapping to treat reflux esophagitis*

Nitro-Bid / *nitroglycerin / antianginal* / D

Nitrodisc / nitroglycerin / *patch* / D

Nitro-Dur / nitroglycerin / *patch* / D

nitrofurantoin / *urinary bacteriostatic* / D

nitrogen mustard / mechlorethamine / *alkylating antineoplastic* / D

nitroglycerin / *coronary vasodilator / antianginal* / D

Nitrol ointment / nitroglycerin / *antianginal* / D

Nitrostat / nitroglycerin / *antianginal* / D

Nizoral / ketoconazole / *topical antifungal* / D

NKA / no known allergies

NKDA / no known drug allergies

nocturia / *urination at night, especially excessively*

nodal (Cardio) / *pertaining to atrioventricular node*

Nolex LA / guaifenesin and phenylpropanolamine / (name changed to Exgest LA in 1994) / *decongestant / expectorant* / D

Nolvadex / tamoxifen / *antineoplastic / for advanced postmenopausal breast cancer* / D

No-Man's Land (Ortho)

nonanion gap metabolic acidosis

noncolicky

non-Q

nontender

Additional Entries

nonsteroidal

nonsteroidal / NSAID / *anti-inflammatory drug* / D

Nordette-28 / *oral contraceptive* / D

Norel / *decongestant* / *antihistamine* / D

Norethin / *oral contraceptive* / D

Norflex / orphenadrine citrate / *skeletal muscle relaxant for injection* / D

norfloxacin / *broad-spectrum bactericidal antibiotic* / D

Norgesic Forte / orphenadrine, aspirin and caffeine / *skeletal muscle relaxant* / D

Norinyl / *oral contraceptive* / D

Norlestrin / *oral contraceptive* / D

normal glandularity (Gyn) / *breast*

normal-pressure (Neuro)

normo- / *normal* / *usual*

normochromic

normocyte/-ic

Normodyne / *antihypertensive* / D

normotensive / *normal arterial blood pressure*

normotopia/-ic / *in the normal location*

Noroxin / norfloxacin / *broad-spectrum antibiotic* / D

Norpace / disopyramide / *antiarrhythmic* / D

Norplant / *five-year birth control* / *wicks placed in arm*

Norpramin / desipramine / *antidepressant* / D

nortriptyline / Aventyl / Pamelor / *antidepressant* / D

Norvasc / amlodipine / *antianginal* / *antihypertensive* / D

nosocomial pneumonia

Novafed / *nasal decongestant* / D

Novocain / procaine / *injection* / *local anesthetic* / D

Novolin L / Novolin N / Novolin R / Novolin 70/30 / *insulin* / D

Now / *action to be initiated within one hour*

Additional Entries

____

____

____

____

noxious stimuli / *hurtful*
NPH insulin / neutral protamine Hagedorn (insulin)
NQMI / non-Q (wave) myocardial infarction
NSAIDs / nonsteroidal anti-inflammatory drugs
NSR / normal sinus rhythm
N-Terminal
Nubain / nalbuphine hydrochloride / *injection* / *narcotic analgesic* / D
nucha / *nape of neck*
nuchal / *pertaining to back of neck* / *rigidity* / *stiff neck*
nucl-, nucleo- / *nucleus* / *nuclear*
nuclear sclerosis
nucleoid
nucleolar pattern
nucleus pulposus (Ortho) / *soft central portion of intervertebral disk* / *gelatinous* / *mass*
nulligravida (Gyn) / *never having been pregnant*
nulliparous (Gyn) / *never having given birth to a child*
nummular / *round, flat, disk shape* / *arranged like a stack of coins* / (in thick mucous sputum)
nutation / nutatory / *nodding, especially involuntary* / *swaying*
Nutraderm / *emollient* / D
Nutri/System / *weight control system*
N&V / nausea and vomiting
Nylen maneuver / *test for benign positional vertigo* / T
Nyquil / *antitussive* / *decongestant* / D [OTC]
nystagmus (Oph) / *eyeballs that rotate back and forth rhythmically*
nystatin / *antifungal* / D
Nytol / *antihistaminic sleep aid* / D [OTC]

Additional Entries

oat cell carcinoma / *a form of carcinoma in which cells
    resemble oat grains*

O

OB-Gyn / obstetrics (and) gynecology

obelion / *a point on the skull*

Ober test (Ortho) / *measuring degree of abduction contrac-
    ture*

objective swelling

obsessed

obstipation / *intractable constipation*

obstruction

obtund/-ent / *easing pain / blunting pain*

obturation/-or / *obstruction*

occipital / *pertaining to the occipital bone at the back of
    the head*

occiput / *back of head*

Occlusal / salicylic acid (discontinued 1994)/ *topical keratolytic* / D

OcuCaps / *vitamin/mineral supplement* / D [OTC]

Occu-Hist (Oph) / *topical antihistamine for eyes* / D

ochronosis / *discoloration*

Octopus (Oph) / *instrument*

Ocufen (Oph) / *ocular nonsteroidal anti-inflammatory* / D

ocular convergence(Oph)

oculgyria/-ic (Oph) / *eyeball rotation*

Ocuvite / *vitamin/mineral supplement* / D

OD / overdose

od / OD (Oph) / L. *oculus dexter / right eye*

Oddi, sphincter of / *sheath of muscle fibers traversing the wall of
    the duodenum*

O-desmethylvenlafaxine

odont- / *tooth*

odontoid

Additional Entries

____

____

____

____

odontoprisis / bruxism / *grinding one's teeth*
odyn-, odyno- / *pain* / e.g., **odyno**phagia
odynophagia / *pain on swallowing*
ofloxacin / Floxin / *broad-spectrum bactericidal antibiotic* / D
Ogen / estropipate / *hormone replacement therapy for postmeno-*
    pausal disorders / D
ogival / *the palate*
-oid / *like* / *resembling* / *form of*
olecranon (Ortho) / *elbow*
olfaction (ENT) / *the sense of smell*
olfactory (ENT) / *relating to the sense of smell*
olig-, oligo- / *a few* / *a little* / *too few* / *too little*
oligemia / *decreased volume of blood*
oligodendroglioma / *tumor*
oligomenorrhea (Gyn)
oligopontocerebellar
oligospermia / *too few sperm cells*
oliguria/ic / *diminished urine*
Ollier disease / *enchondromatosis* / *proliferation of cartilage cells*
    of several bones, causing distortion of growth in length
-ologist / *specialist in the study of* / e.g., bi**ologist**
-ology / *study of (science of) a subject, organ, or a field* /
    e.g., anesthesi**ology**
-oma / *pl.* **omata** / **-omat-** / *a tumor* / *swelling* / *mass of new tissue*
    growth / e.g., my**oma** / *tumor containing muscle tissue*
ombudsman
omentum (GI) / *a fold of peritoneum*
omeprazole / Prilosec / *gastric acid inhibitor* / D
Omniflox / *broad-spectrum antibiotic* / D
omphalic / *pertaining to the umbilicus*
omphalitis / *inflammation of the navel*

Additional Entries

____

____

____

____

oncolysis / *destruction of tumor cell / reduction of swelling or mass*

oncotic pressure / *pressure caused by edema or swelling*

Oncovin (Onc) / vincristine sulfate / *antineoplastic for lung and breast cancer* / D

onlay / *graft laid on*

onset, adult / *in diabetes, disease of adulthood*

onych-, onycho- / *fingernail / toenail*

onychocryptosis / *ingrown toenail*

onychogryphosis / onychogryposis / *enlargement, thickening and increased curvature of fingernails or toenails*

onychomadesis / *shedding of fingernails*

onychomycolysis / *losing a nail due to fungus*

onychomycosis / *nail fungus*

onychoschizia / *horizontal splitting of nails*

oophorectomy / *removal of ovary*

oophor-, oophoro- / *ovary*

oophoritis / *inflammation of an ovary*

O&P / ova & parasites

opacification / *the development of opacity, as of the cornea or lens*

opacities

openia / *decreased*

operculum / *lid or covering structure*

OPG / OPPG / (ocular) oculopneumoplethysmography

-opia / *vision* / e.g., my**opia**

ophiasis (Derm) / *alopecia / hair loss*

ophthalm- / ophthalmo- / *eye / eyes*

ophthalmodynamometry (Oph)

ophthalmologic (Oph)

ophthalmoplegia (Oph)

ophthalmovascular (Oph) / *relating to blood vessels in the eye*

Additional Entries

____

____

____

____

opisth-, opistho- / *backward* / *behind* / e.g., **opisth**otic
opisthion / *a craniometric landmark*
opisthotic / *located behind the ear* / *located in the interior ear*
opisthotonos / *type of spasm*
OPPG / OPG / oculopneumoplethysmography
opponens / *opposing*
opponensplasty, Huber
opponens weakness
opt- / *seeing* / *vision* / *light* / e.g., **opt**ical
optic neuritis (Oph)
Opticrom (discontinued 1993) / *eye drops* / *ocular antiallergic* / D
Optimine / azatadine maleate / *antihistamine* / D
OptiPranolol (Oph) / metipranolol / *drops* / *topical antiglaucoma agent* / D
Optised (Oph) / phenylephrine and zinc sulfate / *eye drops* / *topical ocular decongestant* / *antiseptic* / D
-or / *action* / *state* / *condition* / e.g., vig**or**
    also *person* / e.g., doct**or**, facilitat**or**
Orabase / *mucous membrane anesthetic* / D
Orajel / *topical oral anesthetic* / D
oral gold
oral iron
Orap / pimozide / *antipsychotic* / D
Orasone / prednisone / *glucocorticoid* / *anti-inflammatory* / D
orbicular / *rounded*
orbitopathy / Graves orbitopathy (Oph) / *in Graves disease* / *disease of eyeball*
orchi-, orchio- / *pertaining to the testes*
orchialgia / orchiodynia / *pain in the testis*
orchiectomy / *excision of one or both testes*
orchiodynia / orchialgia / *pain in the testis*

Additional Entries

Oretic / hydrochlorothiazide / *diuretic* / *antihypertensive* / D
Organidin elixir / *for cough control* / *expectorant* / D
organomegaly / *enlargement of the viscera*
organophosphate / *phosphate turned into glucose or sorbitol*
orifice / *entrance* / *outlet*
Orinase / tolbutamide / *antidiabetic* / D
Ornade Spansules / *decongestant* / *antihistamine* / D
oro- / *the mouth*
oropharynx / *part of the pharynx near the soft palate*
orth-, ortho- / *straight* / *normal* / *in proper order* /
   e.g., **ortho**pedic
Ortho All-Flex / *diaphragm*
Ortho-Cept / *birth control pills* / D
Ortho-Cyclen / *birth control pills* / D
Ortho-Novum 7/7/7 / *birth control pills* / D
orthophoria (Oph)
orthopnea/-ic / *breathing discomfort*
orthostatic (Ortho) / *erect posture*
orthostasis / *standing erect*
orthotic/-ics (Ortho) / *making orthopedic appliances*
Ortho Tri-Cyclen / *oral contraceptive* / D
Ortolani sign (Ortho) / *in congenital hip dislocation*
Orudis / ketoprofen / *nonsteroidal anti-inflammatory* / D
Oruvail / ketoprofen / *nonsteroidal anti-inflammatory* / D
os, pl. **ossa** / *bone* / *orifice* / *mouth*
os calcis (Ortho) / *heel bone*
os cervix (Ortho) / *neck bone*
Os-Cal 250/500 / calcium carbonate / *dietary calcium supplement* / D
OS / L. *oculus sinister* (Oph) / *left eye* / *left side*
oscillometry / *the measurement of oscillations, as arteries accom-*
   panying the heartbeat

Additional Entries

Osgood-Schlatter disease (Ortho) / *osteochondrosis of the tibia*
-osis / *condition or disease*
Osler-Weber-Rendu / *telangiectasia* / *dilation of blood vessels*
osmolality / *concentration of a solution expressed in osmoles of solute particles per kilogram of solvent*
osmolarity / *concentration of osmotically active particles in solution, as in urine*
os peroneum (Ortho) / *flexes foot*
ost- / *bone*
oste-, oss-, ossi, -osse- / *-osseous* / *-osteal* / *bony ossicle* / *small bone*
osteitis condensans (Ortho) / *condensing inflammation of bone*
osteitis symphysis pubis (Ortho) / *sclerosis of the pubic bones*
osteoarthritis (Ortho) / *joint disease*
osteoarthrosis (Ortho) / osteoarthritis
osteocartilaginous, extoses (Ortho)
osteochondritis, dissecans (Ortho) / *splitting of pieces of cartilage into the joint*
osteodystrophy (Ortho) / *defective bone formation*
osteogenesis (Ortho) / *formation and development of the bones*
osteoid (Ortho) / *pertaining to bone* / *resembling bone* / *newly formed bone matrix before calcification*
osteoid osteoma (Ortho) / *benign tumor in young bone*
osteoma (Ortho) / *benign, slow-growing mass of mature bone, usually generated in the skull or mandible*
osteomalacia (Ortho) / *disease* / *gradual softening and bending of bone*
osteo-onychial (Ortho) / *pertaining to inflammation of the matrix of a nail, leading to loss of the nail*
osteopenia (Ortho) / *decreased calcification or density* / *decreased bone mass*

Additional Entries

---

osteophyte/-s (Ortho) / *bony growth or protuberance*
osteopoikilosis (Ortho) / *sclerotic foci in the ends of long bones*
osteoporosis (Ortho) / *"brittle bone" disease / affects bone density and strength*
osteotomy(Ortho) / *surgical removal of a bone*
ostium / *door / opening*
-ostomy / *create opening / mouth / passage between organs*
os trigonum (Ortho) / *heel bone*
otitis, externa, media (ENT)
otolaryngology/-ist (ENT) / *pertaining to diseases of the ear and the larynx*
-otomy / *cut into / explore / drain / remove foreign bodies*
otorhinolaryngology/-ist (ENT) / *pertaining to diseases of the ear, nose, larynx and related structures of the head and neck*
otosclerosis / *new growth of bone that causes deafness*
OU / ou / L. *oculi uterque* (Oph) / *each eye*
ou / L. *oculi unitas* / *both eyes*
-ous / *full of / having* / e.g., fam**ous**, danger**ous**, osse**ous**
outliers / *isolated high blood sugars*
outrigger splint
ova-, ovi-, oo-, ovo- / *egg*
ova and parasites
ovalocyte / elliptocyte / *elliptical red blood corpuscle*
ovari-, ovario-, oo-, oophor- / *ovary*
Ovcon-35 / *contraceptive* / D
Ovral / *oral contraceptive* / D
oxa- / *denotes the presence of oxygen*
oxacillin / *antibacterial* / D
oxalate / *a salt of oxalic acid*
oxazepam / Serax / *anxiolytic* / D

Additional Entries

____

____

____

____

Oxepam / *anxiolytic* / *minor tranquilizer* / D
oximeter/-try / *device used to measure photoelectrically the
    oxygen saturation in a blood sample*
Oxipor VHC / *coal tar* / *topical antipsoriatic antiseborrheic* / D [OTC]
Oxistat cream / oxiconazole nitrate / *topical antifungal* / D
oxy- / *in chemistry, denotes the presence of oxygen*
Oxy 10 / benzoyl peroxide / *topical keratolytic* / *for acne* / D
oxybutynin / Ditropan / *anticholinergic* / *urinary antispasmodic* / D
oxycodone / *narcotic analgesic* / D
oxylalia / *speaking fast*
oz / *ounce*

Additional Entries

P/A / P&A / percussion and auscultation
Pabalate / *analgesic / anti-inflammatory* / D
PAC / Platinol, Adriamycin and cyclophosphamide / *chemo-
    therapy protocol*
pacchionian depressions / *in skull*
pachy- / *thick*
pachydermoperiostosis (Derm) / *thickening and deep folds
    and furrows of the skin / in adolescent males*
PA&E / present, active and equal
Paget disease / *breast cancer involving the nipple and
    areola*
pagophagia / *compulsive and frequent eating of ice*
PAH / pulmonary artery hypertension
PAHVC / pulmonary alveolar hypoxic vasoconstriction
palatable / *pleasing to the palate or taste*
palate / palatal / *the palate / roof of the mouth*
palliate/-ion/-ive / *to relieve without curing*
palindromic / *returning / recurrent*
PA line (Radiol) / posteroanterior l.
palmar and dorsal aspect
palpate/-ion / *feeling the body with the hand to examine*
palpebra/ (pl.) -ae (Oph) / *eyelid(s)*
    e.g., inferior p. / *lower eyelid;* superior p. / *upper eyelid*
palpitations (Cardio) / *forceful or irregular heartbeats*
palsy, seventh nerve / *nervus facialis / paralysis or paresis*
Pamelor / nortriptyline / *antidepressant* / D
pan- / *all / entire*
Panafil / *ointment / topical enzyme for wound debridement, wound
    deodorant* / D
pancarditis (Cardio) / *inflammation of the heart*
Pancoast tumor (Pulm) / *pulmonary sulcus tumor*

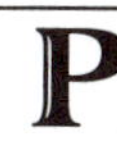

Additional Entries

____
____
____
____

Pancof HC syrup / Robitussin / *antitussive* / D
Pancrease / pancrelipase / *digestive enzymes* / D
pancreate-, pancreatico-, panreato-, pancreo- / *the pancreas*
pancreaticoduodenectomy / pancreatoduodenectomy / *surgical removal of all or part of the pancreas and the duodenum*
pancytopenia / *significant reduction in all types of white blood cells and platelets in the blood*
panendoscopy
panhypopituitarism / *inadequate secretion of all anterior pituitary hormones*
Panoxyl / *bar soap* / *topical keratolytic* / *for acne*
pannus (Oph) / *vascularization of the cornea by granulation tissue*
panus / *inflamed lymphatic gland*
Pap / PAP (Gyn) / *Papanicolaou smear* / *test* / *surveillance* / T
Papanicolaou smear (Gyn) / *Pap/PAP smear/test* / T
papaverine hydrochloride / *vasodilator* / D
papilla / *nipple* / *nipplelike process* / *teat*
papilledema (Oph) / *edema of optic disk*
papilloma / (*pl.*) papillomata / *benign branching tumor*
Papineau grafting (Ortho)
papulo- / *papule* / *pimple* / *pustule*
papular erythematous
papule / *pimple* / *pustule*
papulosquamous / *scaly pimple*
papulovesicular / *an eruption of papules and vesicles*
para- / *beside* / *beyond normal* / *near* / *wrong* / *disordered* / *side by side*
para-aortic (Cardio)
para [2], gravida [2] (Gyn) / *two births, two pregnancies*
paracalcaneal (Ortho) / *heel*
paracentesis / *removing fluid with a fine needle or other instrument*

Additional Entries

____

____

____

____

paraffin section
Paraflex / chlorzoxazone / *skeletal muscle relaxant* / D
Parafon Forte DSC / chlorzoxazone / *skeletal muscle relaxant* / D*
parainfluenza
parakeratosis (Derm)
parallax / *the apparent displacement of an observed object due to the difference between two points of view*
paralumbar (Ortho)
paralysis / *inability to voluntarily move a muscle(s)*
parameters / *variables used to measure or evaluate / determining factor / characteristic*
paramnesia (Neuro) / *memory distortion in which an individual confuses fact and fantasy*
paraneoplastic neuropathy / *metastases / changes in tissue remote from a tumor*
paranesthesia / *anesthesia of lower half of body*
paraparesis / *significant weakness in lower extremities*
paraprotein / *monoclonal immunoglobulin of blood plasma*
parapsoriasis en plaques (Derm)
parasagittal
paraspinous
parathormone / *parathyroid hormone*
parathyroidectomy
paratripsis / *rubbing / chafing*
paraventricular
paravertebral / *alongside a vertebra / alongside the vertebral column*
paregoric / camphorated tincture of opium / D
parenchyma / *the specific cells of a gland or organ*
parenchymal/-matous

Additional Entries

____

____

____

____

parenteral/-ally / *introducing nutrients or medications through means other than the gastrointestinal tract* / i.e., intravenous, intraorbital, subcutaneous

paresis / *partial paralysis*

paresthesia / *tingling of skin* / *abnormal sensation*

paretic / *pertaining to paresis*

parietal / *pertaining to the wall of any cavity*

parietitis / *inflammation of wall*

parieto-occipital / *pertaining to the parietal and occipital bones*

Parinaud (Oph)

paristalsis...**NO!** (see "peristalsis")

Parlodel / bromocriptine mesylate / *antiparkinsonian* / *lactation preventative* / D

Parnate / tranylcypromine sulfate / *antidepressant* / D

paronychia (pronounced "paro-neechia") / *fingernail*

parosteal / *outer surface of periosteum* / *connective tissue covering all bones of the body*

parosteitis (Ortho) / *inflammation of tissue adjacent to bone*

parotid gland / *salivary gland at the base of each ear*

parotitis / *inflammation of parotid gland*

parous / *pertaining to "parity," having given birth*

paroxysm/-mal / *sudden outburst* / *spasm* / *convulsion*

pars, (pl.) partes / *a part* / *a portion* / *division*

pars space (Ortho) / *in spine*

parvus / *small*

PASA (Ortho) / para-aminosalicylic acid

past pointing / *finger-to-nose test*

patella/-ae (n.) (Ortho) / *kneecap*

patellar (adj.) (Ortho)

patellarum (Ortho)

patellofemoral (Ortho) / *pertaining to the patella and the femur*

Additional Entries

____

____

____

____

patent/-cy (pronounced "**pay**-tent") / *open* / *unobstructed* / *exposed*

patent ductus

patent foramen ovale (Cardio)

path-, -pathy, patho-, path•ic / *disease* / *suffer* / *feel*

pathogen / *any organism or substance that causes disease*

pathognomonic / *a sign or symptom on which a diagnosis can be made*

Patrick (Neuro) / T

patulent inflammation

patulous / *pertaining to "patent," being open or exposed*

Pavabid capsulets / *cerebral and peripheral vasodilator* / D

paucity / *smallness* / *insufficiency of number or amount*

Pavlik harness (Ortho)

P-axis

Paxil / paroxetine / *antidepressant* / *for panic disorder* / D

p.c. / L. *post cibum* / *after meals*

pcg / ml

pCO_2, pO_2

PCR / protein catabolic rate

PDA / patent ductus arteriosus

PD / pediatric dose

peau d'orange (Derm) / *skin like an orange*

pectoralis / pectoral / *pertaining to the chest* / *breast bone*

pectus excavatum / *hollow breast*

ped-, pedi-, pedo- / *child* / *foot* / *feet*

pedal (pronounced "**pee**-dal") / *foot pulse*

pedal edema

pedal pulses

Pediamycin / D

pediatrician / *children's physician*

Additional Entries

____

____

____

____

Pediazole / erythromycin and sulfisoxazole / *antibiotic* / D
pedicel (Pod) / *foot / footplate*
pedicel tip amputation (Pod)
pedicles / *footlike structures*
pediculosis pubis / *infestation with lice, especially in pubic hair*
pedis (Pod) / *relating to the foot*
peduncle/-ulated / *tumor on a stalk*
PEEP / positive end expiratory pressure
PEG / pneumoencephalogram
Pel-Epstein / *temperature curve*
peliosis / (syn.) purpura / *condition characterized by hemorrhaging*
Pelligrini-Stieda / *disease*
pellucid / *translucent*
Pemphigoid (Derm) / *blistering*
pemphigus (Derm) / *skin disease* / e.g., p. cicatricial; p. foliaceus
penbutolol sulfate / Levatol / *antiadrenergic* / D
-penia / *decrease / deficiency / insufficiency*
penicillamine / *antirheumatic / metal chelating agent* / D
penicillin benzathine (changed to penicillin V benzathine) / D
Penrose drain / *a soft, thin rubber tube for fluid drainage*
Pentam / pentamidine isethionate / *injection / antiprotozoal* / D
Pentasa / mesalamine / *for ulcerative colitis / for proctitis* / D
Pentolair (Oph) / *eye drops / mydriatic / cycloplegic* / D
Pentothal / thiopental sodium / *general anesthetic* / D
pentoxifylline / Trental / *vasodilator / hemorheologic agent* / D
penumbra / *partial shadow surrounding the complete shadow of
    an opaque object*
Pen•Vee K / phenoxymethyl penicillin / *bactericidal antibiotic* / D
Pepcid / famotidine / *acid controller / for heartburn and acid
    indigestion* / D
Pepsi Cola

Additional Entries

162

Pepto-Bismol / *antidiarrheal* / *antinauseant* / D [OTC]
per- / *throughout* / *through* / *thoroughly* / *excessively*
Percocet / oxycodone and acetaminophen / *narcotic analgesic* / D
Percodan / oxycodone and aspirin / *narcotic analgesic* / D
Percogesic / acetaminophen and phenyltoloxamine / *antihistamine* / *analgesic* / D
percuss / *to perform percussion*
percussible
percussion and auscultation / *in lung exam, tapping on chest (percussion), and listening to responding sounds (auscultation)*
percutaneous / *passed through the skin*
per diem / *by the day*
Perdiem / psyllium / *laxative* / D
perennial, rhinitis / *nonseasonal allergic rhinitis*
perfusate / *the fluid used for perfusion*
perfuse / *to force blood or other fluid to flow over or through an organ or tissue*
perfusion / *the act of perfusing*
peri- / *around* / *about* / *surrounding* / *enclosing* / *covering*
Periactin / cyproheptadine / *antihistamine* / D
periareolar (Gyn) / *near the nipple*
perianal / *surrounding the anus*
periaortic (Cardio) / *surrounding or next to the aorta*
periapical / *around or adjacent to the root of a tooth*
periarteritis nodosa / *arterial inflammation*
periarticular / *surrounding a joint*
peribronchial / *surrounding bronchus or bronchi*
pericallosal (Neuro) / *around white matter in the cerebral hemisphere*

P

Additional Entries

____

____

____

____

pericarditis / *inflammation of the pericardium*
pericaval / *around the superior or inferior vena cava*
perichondrium / *connective tissue membrane around cartilage*
Peri-Colace / docusate and casanthranol / *laxative / stool softener* / D
Peridex / chlorhexidine gluconate / *antimicrobial / for gingivitis* / D
Peridium / D
perihilar / *around the hilum of an organ* / e.g., pulmonary hilar
perihilar calcifications
perimenopausal (Gyn) / *period prior to menopause when estrogen levels naturally decline*
perinatal / *period during or just after birth*
perineal candidiasis (Gyn) / *a form of vaginitis*
perineum / *area between thighs, from the coccyx to the pubis*
perioperative / *near the time of operation*
perioral / *around the mouth*
periorbital (Oph) / *situated around the eye socket*
periosteal (Ortho)
periostitis (Ortho)
peripheral vascular disease / PVD
peristalsis / *progressive, involuntary wavelike movement of muscle, especially in the alimentary canal* / bowel movement
peristasis / *standing still / environment*
peritheliomatous / *pertaining to blood vessel cytoma*
perithoracic / *surrounding or encircling the thorax*
peritoneoscopic / *examination of the peritoneal cavity by an instrument inserted through the abdominal wall*
peritonitis / *inflammation of the peritoneum*
peritracheal / *pertaining to the trachea*
Peritrate SA / *antianginal* / D
periumbilical / *near or around the umbilicus*
periungual / *around the nail*

Additional Entries

Permapen / penicillin G benzathine / *bactericidal antibiotic* / D

pernicious / *harmful* / *tending to cause death or serious injury*

PERL / pupils equal (and) reactive (to) light

PERLA / pupils equal (and) reactive (to) light (and) accommodation

peroneus brevis / *muscle*

peroneal (Ortho) / *pertaining to the fibular area, leg and muscles*

Perphenazine / amitriptyline / *antipsychotic* / *antiemetic* / *intractable hiccough relief* / D

per primam intentionem / *healing*

Persa-Gel / *topical keratolytic* / D

Persantine / dipyridamole / *antiplatelet agent* / D

per se / *in, of, or by itself or oneself* / *intrinsically*

perseverate/-ion / *patient answers a question correctly but gives the same answer to succeeding questions* / *constant repetition of meaningless words*

persistent

Perthes disease / *osteochondrosis of the thigh bone*

pertinent

perusal / *looking over*

pes, pedis, (pl.) pedes / *the foot*

pes anserine bursa (Pod)

pes anserinus (Pod)

pessary / *appliance used to support the uterus*

pes planus (Pod) / *flat feet*

PET / positron emission tomography / T

petechia/-ae / *pinpoint red spot*

pétrissage / foulage / *kneading movement in massage*

petrositis / *inflammation of the temporal bone*

Additional Entries

____

____

____

____

Peyronie disease / *scarring of penis causing abnormal curvature*
Pfannenstiel incision / *abdominal*
Pfizerpen / *bactericidal antibiotic for injection* / D
Pfister faucet
PFT / pulmonary function test / T
pg / picogram
pH / *acid-alkaline measure*
PH / past history
phacolysin / phacolytic (Oph) / *an albumin from the lens of the eye* /
    used in treatment of early cataract
-phage, -phagia, -phago, -phagy / *to eat* / *to swallow*
phagocyte/-osis
phakomatosis / phacomatosis / *developmental congenital anomaly*
    involving central nervous system, eye, and skin
phalangeal (Ortho) / *any of the bones of the fingers or toes*
phalanges / phalanx (Ortho) / *digital bone*
Phalen sign / *for detection of carpal tunnel syndrome*
pharmaco- / *drugs*
pharmacokinetic / *pertaining to the reaction of drugs in the body*
pharyngeal / *pertaining to the pharynx*
pharyngitis, candidal
pharyngitis sicca / atrophic pharyngitis
pharynx / *area between oronasal passages and the esophagus*
-phasia / *speech disorder*
Phazyme / simethicone / *antiflatulent* / D [OTC]
phenacopyriene
Phenaphen / *analgesic* / *antipyretic* / D
phenazopyridine / *urinary tract analgesic* / D
Phenchlor / *decongestant* / *antihistamine* / D
Phenergan / *antihistamine* / *for motion sickness* / *sleep aid* / D
Phenergan with codeine / *narcotic antitussive* / D

Additional Entries

____
____
____
____

Phen/fen / *diet drug* / D
phenobarbital / *anticonvulsant* / *hypnotic* / *sedative* / D
phenol / *topical antiseptic* / *antipruritic* / *local anesthetic* /D
phenolphthalein / *stimulant laxative* / D
phenomenon / (pl.) phenomena
phenothiazine / *antipsychotic* / D
phentermine / *anorexiant* / D
phenylalanine / *essential amino acid*
phenylbutazone / *antirheumatic* / *anti-inflammatory* / D
phenylephrin / *nasal decongestant* / *ocular vasoconstrictor* / D
phenylketonuria / PKU
phenylpropanolamine / *vasoconstrictor* / *nasal decongestant* / D
phenytoin / Dilantin / *anticonvulsant* / D
pheochrome / *certain embryonic cells that stain darkly with
   chromium salts*
pheochromoblast / *embryonic structures that develop into
   pheochrome cells*
pheochromocytoma / *benign encapsulated vascular tumor of the
   adrenal medulla*
pH (*high*) / *acid/alkaline measure*
PHH / posthemorrhagic hydrocephalus
philtrum / *groove in upper lip, below nose*
phimosis / *tightness of foreskin*
pHisoDerm / *soap-free therapeutic skin cleanser*
pHisoHex / hexachlorophene / *bacteriostatic skin cleanser*
phleb-, phlebo- / *vein*
phlebitic/-is / *pertaining to inflammation of a vein*
phlebolith / *stone in vein*
phlebotomy/-ies / *surgical removal of a vein*

P

Additional Entries

____

____

____

____

phlegmasia / *severe inflammation* / e.g., p. alba dolens / *milk leg* / *extreme swelling in leg after childbirth*

phlegmon / *cellulitis*

phlogistic / *pertaining to or inducing inflammation*

phob- / *fear*

-phobe / *one who fears intensely or illogically* / e.g., xeno**phobe** / *one who is abnormally fearful of strangers or foreigners*

phobia / *an intense, abnormal, or illogical fear of a specified thing*

-phobia / *to have intense, abnormal, or illogical fear of a specified thing* / e.g., claustro**phobia** / *fear of being hemmed in, closed in, as in a small room or a crowd*

Phoma / *fungi that are common laboratory contaminants and common plant pathogens*

-phoma / *an allergen*

phon-, phono- / *sound* / *speech* / *voice sounds*

phonating / *uttering*

phonocardiogram

phor-, phoro- / *carrying* / *bearing* / e.g., **phor**esis

Phosamax...**NO!** (see "Fosamax") / D

Phosphaljel (discontinued 1994, no longer labeled for use as an antacid) / D

phosphatase / *enzyme* / T

phospholipid

phosphorus / T

phosphorylase / *enzyme*

photophobia / *abnormal sensitivity to light / extreme fear and avoidance of light*

photoplethysmography

photopleurogram

phren- / *diaphragm / mind / seat of emotions*

-phrenia- / *mental disorder* / e.g, schizo**phrenia**

Additional Entries

Phrygian cap
phthisis / *wasting away*
phylaxis / *the active defense of the body against infection*
phyllo- / **leaf** / **leaflike**
phyllodes / *tumors which show a leaflike structure on being sectioned*
physi-, physio- / *physical* / *physiological* / *natural*
physiatrist/-try / *doctor who specializes in physical medicine*
physo- / *swelling* / *inflating*
phyt-, phyto- / *plants*
phytobezoar / *food ball* / *a gastric food concretion*
phytohemagglutinin / PHA / *a lectin isolated from the red kidney bean*
phytosis / *infection from a vegetable organism*
pi / *16th letter of the Greek alphabet* / *symbol for circumference of a circle* / *symbol for osmotic pressure*
picogram / pg
piano key maneuver
PIC line / *peripherally inserted catheter (line)*
pica / *compulsive eating of dirt, hair, and other items*
pickwickian syndrome / *obese* / *from the description of the fat boy in Dickens' "Pickwick Papers"* / *decreased pulmonary function, and polycythemia*
pico- / *small*
picolinate, chromium / *vitamin*
PID / pelvic inflammatory disease
PIE / pulmonary interstitial emphysema
Pierre Robin syndrome / *cleft palate*
pig bronchus
pigment / *coloring matter or substance* / *any substance whose presence in the tissues or cells of animals or plants colors them*

Additional Entries

____

____

____

____

pigmentalic
pigmenturia / *color in urine*
pignotic
pigtail catheter
pilar / pilary / hairy
pill-rolling tremor / *parkinsonian tremor of the hand*
pilo- / *hair*
pilocarpine / *alkaloid*
pilocarpine (Oph) / *eye drops* / *antiglaucoma agent* / D
piloerection / *erection of hair*
pilonidal / *tuft of hairs in a cyst or sinus opening on skin*
pilos / *hairy*
pimozide / *tranquilizer* / *antipsychotic* / D
Piña colada / *a drink*
pindolol / *vasodilator* / *antiadrenergic* / D
pinguecula (Oph) / *connective tissue that thickens conjunctiva in eye, especially in old age*
pinna (Oto) / *ear*
pioglitazone / *antidiabetic* / D
PIP / proximal interphalangeal (joint) / *joint nearest the hand or foot*
piperacillin / *bactericidal antibiotic* / D
piperonyl butoxide / *pediculicide* / D
pirbuterol acetate / Maxair / *aerosol inhaler* / D
piriform / *pear-shaped*
piriformis muscle spasm
piroxicam / Feldene / *antiarthritic* / *nonsteroidal anti-inflammatory* / D
PIS / primary immunodeficiency syndrome
pisotriquetral (Ortho)
pitting edema / *on pressing flesh with tip of finger, depression remains*

Additional Entries

---

pityriasis rosea (Derm) / *exanthematous disease*
Pityrosporon / *fungi*
PKU / phenylketonuria / *severe recessive trait preventable by early restriction of dietary phenylalanine*
plafond (Ortho)
plagiocephaly / *skull malformation* / *lopsided head*
plain Marcaine / *local anesthetic*
plana verruca / *wart on the foot*
plano- / *flat*
planocellular / *flat cells*
plantar / *pertaining to the sole of the foot*
plantar fasciitis
plantar reflexes
plantar wart / plantar verrucae
plantigrade / *foot*
planuria / *urinating from an abnormal passage of the body*
plaque / *fatty build-up in lining of arteries*
Plaquenil / *antimalarial* / *antirheumatic* / D
-plasia / *formation, especially of cells*
plasmacytosis / *the presence of excess plasma cells in blood*
plasmapheresis / *procedure for separating blood plasma and cells*
plasma protamine paracoagulation / PPP
Plasmodium vivax / *bacteria*
plast-, -plasty / *molding* / *shaping* / *plastic repair* / *reconstruction* / *surgical repair of*
platelet / *disc-shaped structure in blood of all mammals*
Platinol / *antineoplastic* / *for testicular, ovarian, bladder, lung, head, neck and esophageal cancers* / D
Plastizote insert (Ortho)
platy- *flat, broad*
platypellic / platypelloid / platypelvic / *wide pelvis*

Additional Entries

____
____
____
____

platypodia / *flatfooted*
Plendil / *antihypertensive* / D
pleocytosis / *increased lymphocytes in spinal fluid*
pleomorphic / polymorphic / *fungi with two or more spore forms*
plethora / *general term denoting a florid complexion* / *specifically, an excessive amount of blood* / *any excess in quantity*
plethysmography / *study of peripheral circulation*
pleur-, pleura-, pleuro- / *rib* / *side* / *membrane covering the chest cavity*
pleuracentesis / thoracentesis / *puncturing the chest wall for aspiration of fluids*
pleura/-al / *pertaining to the membrane surrounding the lungs and lining the walls of the pleural cavity*
pleurisy/-itic / *inflammation of the pleura, usually producing chest pain*
plexitis / *inflammation of a plexus*
plexus, solar / *near the abdomen/celiacus*
plication / *tucks*
plombage / *sealing* / *filling* / *lung treatment*
pluri- / *several* / *more*
pluriresistant / *resistant to several drugs*
Plummer-Vinson syndrome / *cracks or fissures at the corners of the mouth*
plus extensors / minus extensors
PMI / point of maximal intensity / point of maximal impulse
PNAB / percutaneous needle aspiration biopsy
PND / paroxysmal nocturnal dyspnea
-pnea, pneo- / *breathing* / *respiration*
pneum- / *lung* / *air* / *also* ... **pneumat-** / *relating to air or respiration*
pneumatosis cystoides intestinalis pneumococcus/-i/-al

Additional Entries

____

____

____

____

Pneumocystis carinii / *micro-organism that causes inter-stitial plasma cell pneumonia*

pneumomediastinum / *release of air into mediastinal tissues, usually from emphysema or pulmonary rupture*

pneumonectomy / *surgical removal of all pulmonary lobes from a lung*

pneumoniae / *bacteria*

pneumonitis / *lung inflammation*

pneumotachygraph / *instrument for recording the velocity of respired air*

pneumothorax / *presence of air or gas in pleural cavity*

pneumothoraces / *plural of pneumothorax*

Pneumovax / *pneumococcal vaccine* / D

PNT (Cardio) / paroxysmal nodal tachycardia

p.o. / L. *per os* / *by mouth* / *orally*

pod-, podo- / *foot* / *foot-shaped*

podagra / *severe pain in foot* / *gouty pain in great toe*

podophyllin / *caustic, cytotoxic agent* / *for genital warts* / D

-poiesis / *production* / *producing* / *making*

poikilo- / *irregular* / *varied*

poikilocyte / *an irregular shaped red blood cell*

poikilocytosis / *blood erythrocytes that show abnormal variation in shape*

poikilothermy / *when body temperature varies according to environmental temperatures*

poikilothymia / *abnormal variations of mood*

Polaramine / *antihistamine* / D

pole

polio- / *gray* / *gray matter*

pollicis longus brevis / *muscle*

poly- / *many* / *multiple* / *often*

P

Additional Entries

____

____

____

____

polyarticular / multiarticular / *pertaining to many joints*
polyarcuate
polychromasia / *the tendency of certain cells to stain with dyes*
Polycillin / *ampicillin / penicillin-type antibiotic* / D
Polycitra-K crystals / *urinary alkalizing agent*
polyclonal / *proteins from more than a single clone of cells*
polycystic / *made up of many cysts*
polycystic pancreas
polycythemia/-ic / *abnormal increase in red cell mass in blood*
polycythemia vera / *chronic form of polycythemia*
polydipsia / *excessive thirst*
polyethylene
polyhedral / *many sides / many facets*
polyhydramnios / *excess amniotic fluid*
polymenorrhea / *abnormally frequent menstrual cycles*
polymorphonuclear cells / "polys"
polymyalgia / *muscle pain*
polymyalgia rheumatica / *proximal joint and muscle pain, and high sedimentation (sed) rate / usually in the elderly*
polymyositis / *disease of skeletal muscle*
polyparesis
polypectomy / *surgical removal of a polyp*
polyphagia / *excessive hunger*
polypoid lesions
polyposis / *existence of several polyps*
polypropylene brace
polyserositis / *inflammation of serous membranes*
polys / polynuclear neutrophils
Polytrim / *eye drops / ophthalmic antibiotic* / D
polyuria / *excessive urination*
polyvinyl

Additional Entries

pompholyx (Derm) / *skin eruption between the toes and fingers*
Pondimin / *anorexiant* / *central nervous system depressant* / D
Ponstel / mefenamic acid (Gyn) / *for cramps* / D
pontine infarct (Neuro) / *in the pons area of the brain*
poples / popliteal (Ortho) / *posterior surface of knees*
por-, poro- / *pore* / *duct* / *opening*
porcine valve / *graft derived from swine*
porencephalia / porencephaly (Neuro) / *cavities in the infant brain*
pork Lente / *insulin* / D
porokeratosis (Derm) / *rare skin disorder*
porphobilinogen / *immediate precursor of the porphyrins*
porphyria/-phyrin / e.g., p. cutanea tarda hereditaria
porphyrin / *any compound containing the porphyrin structure*
portacaval / *connecting the portal vein and the vena cava*
porta hepatis / hepatic portal
portal vein
Porter-Silber / *plasma*
positive ANA 1:640
POSS / percutaneous on-surface stimulation
post-, postero- / *after* / *behind* / *posterior*
posterior fontanelle / *soft spot in infant's head*
posterior tibial
posteroinferior
postherpetic neuralgia / *pain following attack of shingles*
posthepatic / *behind the liver*
posthitis / *inflammation of prepuce*
postictal / *after seizure or stroke*
postpartum / *after childbirth*
postphlebitic

Additional Entries

____
____
____
____

postprandial / *after meals*
postrotator
post-tussive rales / *rales heard in lungs after coughing has ceased*
postural hypotension / *blood pressure affected by the posture of the body* / e.g, by standing up
potassium / a metallic element (K) / D
potentia / *power*
poudrage / *powder for fusion*
PPD / purified protein derivative (of tuberculin)
PPT Plastagote / *insoles*
praecox / *early*
Pramosone / *cream* / *lubricant* / *ointment* / *topical corticosteroid* / *local anesthetic* / D
Pramoxine / *cream* / *topical local anesthetic* / D
Pravachol / *cholesterol-lowering antihyperlipidemic* / D
pravastatin / Pravachol / *for cholesterol treatment* / D
Praziquantel / *anthelmintic* / *destructive to worms* / D
prazosin / *antihypertensive* / D
pre- / *before* / *in front of*
precipitated
precordia / precordium / antecardium (GI) / *the epigastrium and anterior surface of the lower part of the thorax*
precordial (GI)
Precose / *inhibitor* / *for type II diabetes mellitus* / D
prednisolone / *glucocorticoid* / D
prednisone burst "to off" / *prednisone therapy*
preeclampsia / *toxicity of pregnancy*
preexcitation (Cardio) / *premature ventricular activation*
pregnancy test / *urine*
pregnandiol / D
Premarin 0.625 mg / *estrogen replacement therapy (ERT)*

Additional Entries

---

premonitory / *serving as a warning*
Premphase / estrogens, conjugated / D
Prempro / estrogen / D
prepatellar bursitis
preponderance / *most*
prepuce/-putial / *pertaining to the fold of skin covering the glans penis*
prepyloric / *pertaining to the digestive process*
prerogative / *choice*
presacral
Presalin (discontinued 1995) / *analgesic / anti-inflammatory* / D
presby-, presbyo- / *old age*
presbyastasia / *in old age, motor incoordination with inability to stand*
presbycusis / presbyacusis / *in old age, diminished hearing*
presbyopia / *in old age, diminished eyesight*
pressure palsy / *temporary paralysis due to pressure on a nerve*
PreSun Spray / D
presyncope/-copal / *about to faint*
pretibial / *pertaining to the anterior part of leg and muscles*
preurethritis / *inflammation around urethral orifice of vaginal vestibule*
Prevacid / lansoprazole / *antiulcerative / antisecretory for duodenal ulcer* / D
priapism / *permanent erection*
Prilosec / omeprazole / *for gastroesophageal reflux disease* / D
Primatene Mist / epinephrine / *bronchodilator / for bronchial asthma* / D [OTC]
Primaxin / imipenem/cilastatin / *bactericidal antibiotic* / D
primidone / Mysoline / *anticonvulsant* / D

Additional Entries

PRIND / prolonged reversible ischemic neurologic deficit

Principen / ampicillin / *penicillin-type antibiotic* / D

Prinivil / lisinopril / *antihypertensive / ACE inhibitor / for congestive heart failure / for acute myocardial infarction* / D

Prinzide / lisinopril and hydrochlorothiazide / D

Prinzmetal angina (Cardio) / *chest pain due to spasm of coronary arteries*

p.r.n. / *L. pro re nata / as needed / as the occasion arises*

pro- / *in front of / before / forward*

Probampacin / ampicillin and probenecid / *antibiotic / for gonorrhea* / D

Pro-Banthine / propantheline bromide / *peptic ulcer treatment adjunct / antispasmodic* / D

probenecid / *uricosuric* / D

procainamide / *antiarrhythmic* / D

Procan SR / *antiarrhythmic* / D

procarbazine / *antibiotic antineoplastic* / D

Procardia XL / nifedipine / *antianginal / antihypertensive* / D

procelous / *concave anteriorly*

procidentia / *prolapsed uterus*

proct-, procto- / *anus / anal canal / rectum*

proctalgia fugax / *episodic severe pain in the rectum from spasm of levator and coccygeal muscles*

proctitis / *inflammation of the rectum*

proctocolectomy

Proctocort / hydrocortisone / *anorectal cream / topical corticosteroid* / D

ProctoCream / *anorectal cream / topical corticosteroid* / D

ProctoFoam / *anorectal aerosol foam / topical local anesthetic* / D

proctoscopic

proctosigmoidoscopy

Additional Entries

prodrome / *precursor*
profundaplasty / *reconstruction of an occluded or stenosed deep femoral artery*
Progestasert / progesterone / *intrauterine contraceptive* / D
progesterone in oil / *injection* / *contraceptive* / D
progesterone / *intrauterine contraceptive* / D
prognathic/-nathous / *projecting jaws*
Prograf / *to prevent organ rejection after liver transplant* / D
progressive supranuclear palsy
prolactin / *protein hormone that stimulates milk secretion*
prolactinoma
prolactin testosterone
proliferative / *increasing*
Prolixin / fluphenazine / *antipsychotic* / D
Proloid (discontinued 1992) / *for hypothyroidism* / *for thyroid cancer* / D
Proloprim / trimethoprim / *anti-infective* / *antibacterial*
prometaphase / *a phase of the division of a cell*
promethazine / *antiemetic* / *antihistamine* / D
ProMod / *powder* / *oral protein supplement*
promyelocyte / *a cell in development between myeloblast and myelocyte*
pronation / *turning the palm up or down* / *extending the foot* / *lying prone, face downward*
pronator drift
Pronestyl / procainamide / *antiarrhythmic* / D
propafenone hydrochloride / Rythmol (Cardio) / *antiarrhythmic* / D
Propacet / propoxyphene and acetaminophen / *narcotic analgesic* / D
Propagest / phenylpropanolamine / *nasal decongestant* / *diet aid* / D
Propecia / *for hair growth*
Propine (Oph) / dipivefrin / *eye drops* / *antiglaucoma agent* / D

P

Additional Entries

---

prophylactic/-axis / *prevention/guarding against infection and disease*

propoxyphene / *narcotic analgesic* / D

propranolol / Inderal / *antiarrhythmic* / *migraine preventative* / D

proprioceptive / *receiving stimuli within the tissues of the body*

proptosis/-tic (Oph) / *abnormal protrusion of the eyeball*

Propulsid / cisapride / *for nocturnal heartburn due to gastroesophageal reflux disease (GERD)* / D

propylene glycol / *humectant* / *solvent* / D

propylthiouracil / PTU / *thyroid inhibitor* / D

Proscar / finasteride / *androgen* / *hormone inhibitor* / *for benign prostatic hyperplasia* / D

ProSobee / *hypoallergenic infant formula*

ProSom / estazolam / *sedative* / *hypnotic* / D

prostaglandin / *a component derived from unsaturated fatty acids*

prostate / *male genitalia* / *the prostate gland*

prostatectomy / *surgical removal of prostate*

prostatic acid phosphatase / PAP

prostatic hypertrophy

prostatic specific antigen / PSA

prostatitis / *inflammation of the prostate*

prostatomy / prostatotomy / *incision into the prostate*

ProStep / *nicotine patch*

prosthesis / *an artificial body part*

prosthetic / *pertaining to an artificial part*

prosthodontist / *specialist in artificial teeth or parts of teeth*

protective extension resection

proteinuria / albuminurea / *protein in the urine*

Proteus mirabilis / *bacteria* / *leading cause of urinary infections*

Proteus rettgeri / *bacteria*

pro time / *prothrombin time*

Additional Entries

____

____

____

____

protocol / *plan*
protodiastolic murmur
proton pump inhibitors
protoporphyrin
protriptyline / *tricyclic antidepressant* / D
providencia stuartii / *bacteria* / *the major agent in burn infections*
Proventil inhaler / *bronchodilator* / D
Proventil Repetabs / *bronchodilator* / D
Provera / medroxyprogesterone acetate / *for abnormal uterine bleeding* / D
proximal interphalangeal joint / PIP / *fingers* / *thumb*
Prozac / fluoxetine / *antidepressant* / *treatment for obsessive/compulsive disorder* / D
prune belly disorder / *defective abdominal muscles*
prurigo nodularis (Derm)
pruritus/-tic / *itching* / e.g., p. ani; p. vulva
psammoma / *tumor* / *sandlike material*
PSBO / partial small bowel obstruction
pseud-, pseudo- / *false*
pseudacusis / *sounds heard falsely or imagined*
pseudoaneurysm / *dilatation and tortuosity of a vessel, giving appearance of an aneurysm*
pseudobulbar / *supranuclear paralysis of bulbar nerves*
pseudocyesis / *false pregnancy*
pseudocyst / *accumulation of fluid in cystlike form*
pseudoephedrine / *vasoconstrictor* / *nasal decongestant* / D
pseudohydronephrosis / *cyst near kidney*
pseudohypha/-ae / *fungal cells*
Pseudomonas aeruginosa / *bacteria*
pseudoplegia / *paralysis of hysterical origin*

P

Additional Entries

---

pseudopterygium (Oph)
pseudotumor cerebri (Neuro) / *condition in which brain simulates presence of intracranial tumor*
pseudoxanthoma elasticum (Oph)
psittacosis / *disease from birds of parrot family*
psoai sign / *seen in appendicitis / pain on hyperextension of hip upon contact between inflammatory process and psoas muscle*
psoas / *muscle / loin muscles /* e.g., p. shadow
psomophagia / *the habit of swallowing food without thoroughly chewing it*
Psorcon / *ointment / topical corticosteroid anti-inflammatory*
psoralen with radiation / *photochemotherapy*
psoriasis/-atic/-iform (Derm) / *chronic skin lesions*
psoriasis guttata (Derm)
PSP (Uro) / phenolsulfonphthalein
psych-, psycho- / *the mind / mental / psychological*
   •psychologist / a licensed specialist in clinical psychology
   •psychiatrist / a medical doctor who diagnoses and treats mental disorders and writes prescriptions; M.D. who "heals the mind"
psych / psychiatry
psychogenic itching / *caused by mental factors, not organic factors*
psychotropic / *drugs that affect the mental state*
psyllium / plantago seed / plantain seed / *bulk laxative* / D
pt / patient
PT / prothrombin time
PT / PTT / partial thromboplastin time
PTCA / percutaneous transluminal coronary angioplasty
pterion / *sphenoid bone*
pterygium / pterygoid (Oph)
PTH level / parathyroid hormone (level)

Additional Entries

-ptosis / *falling* / *sagging* / *sinking down* / *drooping*
pubic / *pertaining to or situated near the os pubis*
puborectalis / *pertaining to pubis and rectum*
PUD / pelvic ulcer disease
puddling / *blood pooling in lower extremities*
pudendum / *external genitalia, especially female*
pudendal area / *groin, especially female*
Pudenz button / *in hydrocephalus*
puerperium / *confinement after labor*
pulmo-, pulmon-, pulmono- / *the lungs*
Pulmo-Aide
pulmonary alveolar proteinosis
pulmonic / *pertaining to the lungs* / *pertaining to the pulmonary artery*
pulmozyme / *bronchitis*
pulposus / *pulpy* / *nucleus*
pulsatile / *throbbing* / *beating*
pulse / pulsus / *heart induced rhythmical dilation of an artery, and sometimes, a vein or vascular organ*
pulse ox / pulse oximetry / *oxygen measurement* / T
pulsus paradoxus (Cardio) / *abnormal variations pulse*
punctate / *distinguished by points or dots*
punctate lucencies
punctate rash
punctum
pupillary response (Oph)
puric / *pertaining to pus or purine*
Purkinje's cells / *fibers*
purpura/-ic / *hemorrhage into skin*
purulent / *containing pus* / *forming pus*
pustular

P

Additional Entries

____

____

____

____

pustules / *visible collections of pus in hair follicle or sweat pore*
PUVA treatments (Derm) / psoralen ultraviolet A-range (treatments)
PVC (Cardio) / premature ventricular contraction
PVC, unifocal, cecal
pyarthrosis / suppurative arthritis
pyel-, pyelo- / *pelvis / renal pelvis / kidney*
pyelogram
pyelocaliectasis / caliectasis (Uro) / *dilation of calices (kidney area) / usually due to obstruction or infection*
pyelonephritis (Uro)
pyknodysostosis / *dwarfism*
pyoderma / *any purulent skin disease*
pyloric (GI)
pyloroplasty
pylorospasm
pylorus/-i/-ic (GI) / *muscular sphincter in the stomach*
pyo- / *pus / accumulation of pus*
pyogenic/-genous / *producing pus*
pyorrhea / *discharge of pus*
pylorus / *opening from stomach into duodenum*
pyosalpinx (Gyn)
pyramidal / *any structure shaped like a pyramid*
pyr-, pyreto-, pyro / *fire / fever / heat / hot*
pyrene / *a polycyclic hydrocarbon*
pyrenemia / *condition in which nucleated red blood cells are present*
pyrenie plaque
pyrethrins / *insecticide and topical pediculicide*
pyrethron / *neutral ester from pyrethrum*
pyrethrum / pyrethrin / *flower / chysanthemum*
pyreto- / *fever*
pyretogenous / *causing fever*

Additional Entries

pyrexia / fever
pyribenzamine / tripelennamine / *antihistamine* / D
Pyridiate / *urinary analgesic* / D
Pyridium / *urinary analgesic* / D
pyridoxine / Nestrex / *vitamin B_6* / D
pyro- / *fever* / *fire* / *heat*
pyrogen / *a fever-producing substance*
pyrophosphate crystals / *joint fluid*
pyrosis / *pain or burning sensation when belching* / *heart-burn*
pyruvate / *a salt or ester of pyruvic acid* / e.g., p. kinase
pyuria (GU) / *pus in urine*

P

Additional Entries

____
____
____
____

q. / L. *quaque* / every
q.a.m. / L. *quaque* [a.m.] / every morning
q.d. / L. *quaque die* / every day
q.h. / L. *quaque hora* / every hour
q.12h. / every 12 hours
q.i.d./ L. *quater in die* / four times a day
q.l. / L. *quantum libet* / as much as desired
q.n. / L. *quaque nocte* / every night
q.o.d. / L. *quaque altera die* / every other day
q.o.n. / L. *quaque altera nocte* / every other night
QRS complex
Q-tip
quadrantectomy
quadratus lumborum
quadriceps / *four heads* / *muscles*
quadriparesis / *weakness of all four limbs*
quadriplegia / *paralysis of all four limbs*
quantitative ß-hCG / *pregnancy test* / T
quartile / *a fourth*
Queckenstedt sign / *pertaining to veins in the neck*
Quervain...**NO!** / (see "deQuervain")
Questran Light / *powder* / *adjunct to diet for reduction of elevated serum cholesterol*
Queyrat erythroplasia / *form of epithelial dysplasia*
quiescent / *inactive* / *quiet* / *at rest*
Quinaglute / quinidine / *antiarrhythmic* / D
Quinamm / *for nocturnal leg cramps* / D
quinapril HCl / Accupril / quinapril hydrochloride / *antihypertensive* / *ACE inhibitor* / D
Quincke disease / *angioedema*
Quinidex Extentabs / quinidine / *antiarrhythmic* / D

Additional Entries

____
____
____
____

quinine sulfate / Formula Q / *antiarrhythmic* / D
quinidine (Cardio) / *antiarrhythmic* / D
Quiphile (discontinued 1996) / *for nocturnal leg cramps* / D
Qwell...**NO!** / (see "Kwell")
QVC cream
Q-Vel / *for nocturnal leg cramps* / D

Additional Entries

Raaf catheter
RA / rheumatoid arthritis
RA blood gases / room air (blood gases)
rachi-, rachio-, / *the spine / spinal column / backbone*
rachitic / *pertaining to or affected with rickets*
rachiocampsis / *curvature of the spine*
rachiocentesis / *lumbar puncture*
radial keratotomy / RK (Oph)
radicular / *pertaining to the radic/root*
radiculopathy / *back pain*
radiocontrast (Radiol)
radiographic / *x-ray*
radioimmunoassay / *to determine antibody concentrations*
radioiodine / radioactive isotope of iodine / *treatment of thyroid*
radiolucencies / *radiolucent areas appear dark on x-rays*
radionuclide / *disintegrates with emission of radiation*
radius (Ortho) / *bone on thumb side of forearm*
Raimondi spring catheter
rales (Pulm) / *noises in lungs while breathing*
raloxifene HCL / *drug study / antiestrogen / D*
ramipril / Altace / *antihypertensive / angiotensin-converting
    enzyme inhibitor / D*
Ramsay Hunt syndrome / *facial herpes zoster*
ramus/-i / *a primary division of nerve or blood vessel / nerve
    branches /* e.g., r. marginalis
range-of-motion
ranitidine / Zantac / *treatment of gastrointestinal ulcers / D*
raphe / *line of union of two contiguous structures*
rapid profile II
rarefaction / *becoming less dense*
RAST screen / radioallergosorbent (screen) / T

Additional Entries

____
____
____
____

Raudixin / rauwolfia serpentina (discontinued 1995) / *antihyper-tensive* / D
Raynaud phenomenon / *cold hands*
ray resection
RBBB (Cardio) / right bundle branch block
RBC / red blood cell
RBS / random blood sugar
reactant / *substance in chemical reaction*
recessus / recess / *withdrawing*
recombinant interleukin II
Recombivax HB / *hepatitis B vaccine* / D
recrudescence/-ent / *new outbreak* / *active again*
recruitment (Oto) / *in audiology, perceived loudness of a sound abnormally increased by a slight increase in its intensity*
rect-, recto- / *rectum*
rectal erythema
rectocele (Gyn) / *protrusion or herniation of posterior vaginal wall with anterior wall of rectum through the vagina*
rectorrhaphy / *suture of rectum and anus*
rectosigmoidectomy / *surgical removal of rectum and sigmoid colon*
rectum/-s/ recta / *end portion of digestive tube*
rectus / *muscles*
recumbent / *reclining* / *lying down* / *leaning*
recurrence
recurvation / *bending back*
redound / *to flow back* / *come back* / *have effect or result upon*
reducible
redundancy/-ant
Redux / dexfenfluramine / *for weight control* / D
Reebok / *shoes*
Reed-Sternberg cells / *giant hystiocytic cells, as in Hodgkin disease*

Additional Entries

____

____

____

____

reflexes

refraction / (Physics) *change of direction of a ray of light, sound, heat, or the like* / (Oph) *ability of the eye to refract light so as to form an image on the retina*

refractory / obstinate / *resistant to treatment*

Regitine / papaverine T / *antihypertensive* / *for pheochromocytoma* / D

Reglan / metoclopramide / *antidopaminergic* / *antiemetic for chemotherapy* / D

rehab / rehabilitation

Reid sleeve / *for lymphedema*

Reiter disease / *in young men, triad of urethritis, conjunctivitis and arthritis*

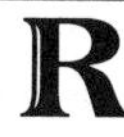

Relafen / nabumetone / *antiarthritic* / *nonsteroidal anti-inflammatory* / D

relevant / pertinent / *pertaining to the matter at hand*

remotely / *long ago*

renal artery stenosis

Rendu-Osler-Weber disease / *hereditary hemorrhagic telangiectasia*

Renova / *retinoid for photodamage and fine wrinkles* / *for age spots and wrinkling* / D

renovascular / *pertaining to or affecting blood vessels of the kidney*

ReoPro / abciximab / *antiplatelet agent* / *prevents clot formation during angioplasty* / D

Replens (Gyn) / *gel* / *vaginal lubricant*

repolarization / *re-establishment of polarity* / *return of cell membrane to resting potential after depolarization*

Rescon-GG / *decongestant* / *expectorant* / D

resection / *excision of all or a portion of an organ or other structure*

reserpine / *rauwolfia derivative* / *antihypertensive* / D

Additional Entries

____

____

____

____

residuum / residua / *remainder*
resin sponge uptake of triiodothyronine
resistant
resisted hip extension, flexion
Resperidol / D
respirations 16, easy / *part of lung exam on physical exam*
rest attenuation
Restoril / temazepam / *sedative* / *hypnotic* / D
resuscitation / *to revive*
Retavase / *thrombolytic for use in myocardial infarction* / D
reticulocyte / *young red blood cell*
retin-, retino- (Oph) / *the retina*
retinaculum / *structure that holds an organ in place*
Retin-A / tretinoin / *topical keratolytic* / *for acne* / D
retinitis pigmentosa (Oph)
retinoschisis (Oph)
retinopathy (Oph)
retro- / *backwards* / *situated behind*
retrocaval (Cardio) / *behind the vein that empties into the right atrium of the heart*
retrogasserian / *trigeminal ganglion on the sensory root of the fifth cranial nerve*
retrolisthesis / retrospondylolisthesis / *congenital defect involving the fifth lumbar vertebra*
retromolar trigone / *pertaining to molar tooth*
retro-orbital (Oph)
retroperitoneal
Retrovir / *antiviral for HIV, AIDS, and AIDs-related complex* / D
Retzius space / *pertaining to retropubic space between bladder and pubic symphysis*
revascularization

Additional Entries

____

____

____

____

Reye syndrome / *sequel of viral upper respiratory disease in childhood / sometimes fatal*
Rezulin / troglitazone / *for diabetes*
Rh / rhesus factor / *of blood*
rhabd-, rhabdo- / *rod-shaped*
Rhabditis / *small nematode worms*
rhabdomyoma / *benign tumor derived from striated muscle*
rhabdomyolysis
rhabdomyosarcoma / *malignant neoplasm*
rhagades / *fissures in skin*
rheoencephalography/-gram / *graphic recording of changes in conductivity of tissue due to vascular factors*
rheumatica / polymyalgia
rheumatology
Rheumatrex / *antirheumatic / antipsoriatic / antineoplastic for leukemia / D*
-rhexis / *break / rupture / burst*
rhin- / *nose*
rhinitis (ENT) / *inflammation of nasal mucous membrane*
Rhinocort / *nasal inhaler / D*
rhinolith / *nasal concretion*
rhinophonia / *nasal tone in speaking*
rhinophyma / brandy nose / *hypertrophy (increase in size) of nose*
rhinorrhea / *watery discharge from nasal mucous membrane*
rhizo- / *root*
rhizotomy / *cutting spinal nerves*
RHM / routine health maintenance
rhomboidal / *shaped like a rhomboid*
rhonchi / rhonchus (Pulm) / *dry rattling in bronchial tube / heard on auscultation / due to partial obstruction*
rhus (Derm) / *dermatitis*

R

Additional Entries

____

____

____

____

-rhythmia / *rhythm*
RIA / radioimmunoassay
RIBA
rib belt
RICE / rest, ice, compression (and) elevation
Richter hernia / *only a portion of the bowel wall is involved*
Rickettsia / *bacteria*
Ridaura / auranofin / gold compound / *antirheumatic* / *for arthritis* /D
Riedel lobe / *thyroiditis*
Rifamate / rifampin and isoniazid / *tuberculostatic* / D
rifampin / *antibacterial* / *antituberculosis treatment* / D
right-hand dominant / right-handed
rigidity, nuchal / *stiff neck* / *back of neck rigidity*
rigor / chill (pronounced "rye-gor")
Rilutek / riluzole / *treatment for amyotrophic lateral sclerosis (ALS)* / D
rima / *cleft* / *crack*
Rinne test (Oto)
Riopan / magaldrate (discontinued 1994) / D [OTC]
RISA cisternogram / *radiography of the basal cistern of the brain*
risperidone / Risperdal / *for psychosis* / D
ristocetin / *antibiotic* / *formerly used for severe staph infection* / D
Ritalin-SR / methylphenidate / *analeptic* / *central nervous system (CNS) stimulant* / *for attention deficit hyperactivity (ADHDs) disorders* / D
ritodrine / *smooth muscle relaxant* / D
rituximab / for non-Hodgkin lymphoma / D
RLL / right lower lobe
RLQ / right lower quadrant
RNP antibody / ribonucleoprotein (antibody)
R/O / rule out

Additional Entries

Robaxin / *skeletal muscle relaxant* / D
Robaxisal / *skeletal muscle relaxant* / *analgesic* / D
Robinul / *anticholinergic/ peptic ulcer treatment adjunct* /D
Robitussin A-C / *narcotic antitussive* / *expectorant* / D
Rocaltrol / *treatment of hypocalcemia in dialysis patients*/D
Rocephin / *antibiotic* / D
Rochalimaea Henselae / *a species of the Rickettsiaceae family that causes bacillary angiomatosis and cat scratch fever*
Rockwood exercises / *upper extremity therapeutic exercise program using Thera-Band*
rocuronium bromide / Zemuron / *skeletal muscle relaxant*/D
roentgen/-ogram / *pertaining to international unit of exposure dose for x-rays or gamma rays*
Roger disease (Cardio) / *ventricular septal defect*
Roho / *specialized bed for care of decubiti*
Rokitansky disease / *a traction diverticulum of the esophagus*
rolandic / EEG / *central sulcus of cerebrum which separates frontal from parietal lobe of brain* / *described by Luigi Rolando*
ROM / range of motion
Romberg sign / *inability to maintain body balance when eyes are shut and feet are close together* / *seen in sensory ataxia* / T
rongeur / *instrument for cutting bone*
rosacea / acne (Derm) / *face*
room air gases
Rorschach test / Ror / RIT / *inkblot test* / T
Rotacaps / *encapsulated powder for inhalation* / D
rotator / *muscle used to turn a body part circularly* / *e.g.,* r. cuff
rote fashion / rote memory
Roth disease / meralgia paresthetica
Rotor syndrome / *chronic familial jaundice*

Additional Entries

____

____

____

____

rouleau/-eaux / *roll of red cells, like roll of dimes*

Roux-en-Y, anastomosis

Rowasa / mesalamine / *in enema* / *for treatment of active ulcerative colitis* / D

Roxanol / morphine sulfate / *narcotic analgesic* / D

Roxicet / oxycodone and acetaminophen / *narcotic analgesic* / D

Roxiprin / oxycodone and aspirin / *narcotic analgesic* / D

RPR / rapid plasma reagent

-rrhagia / *excessive discharge* / e.g., meno**rrhagia**

-rrhaphy / *suture* / e.g., myo**rrhaphy** / *suture of a muscle*

-rrhea / *discharge* / e.g., meno**rrhea**

-rrhexis / *rupture* / e.g., cardio**rrhexis**; angio**rrhexis**

RRR / regular rate (and) rhythm / *in heart exam*

RSO / right salpingo-oophorectomy

RTAZ / *dictation phone system*

RT3U / RT3 Uptake / *resin sponge uptake of triiodothyronine*

rubella / *several types of measles*

rubeola / *measles*

rubeosis / *redness*

Rubin test (Gyn) / *involving fallopian tubes*

rubor / *redness* / *inflammation*

Rubramin PC / *antiemetic* / *vitamin B_{12} supplement* / D

rubra vera (Derm) / *skin redness*

rubrum / *red*

ruga/ (pl.) rugae / *ridge* / *wrinkle or fold* / *especially in mucous membrane* / e.g., r. of stomach; r. of vagina

rule out - R/O

Rumpel-Leede phenomenon / *minute subcutaneous hemorrhages on upper arm, below where tourniquet had been applied for ten minutes*

RURTI / recurrent upper respiratory tract infection

Additional Entries

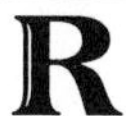

rush / *a powerful wave of contractile activity traveling long distances down the small intestine / caused by intense irritation*

Ru-Tuss / guaifenesin and pseudoephedrine / *decongestant / antihistamine* / D

R-Wave

Rx / prescription / therapy

Rynatan / *pediatric decongestant / antihistamine* / D

Rythmol / propafenone / *antiarrhythmic* / D

Additional Entries

____

____

____

____

S_1—S_4 (Cardio) / *first to fourth heart sounds*
S1—S5 / *first to fifth sacral vertebrae or nerves*
saccade (Oph) / *the series of jumps the eyes make in scanning a line of print*
sacculus / *little bag or sac*
sacculated / *pouched*
Sach disease / Tay-Sacks disease / *fatal inherited disease of children, mainly in Jewish populations*
sacral-Ferguson
sacroiliac (Ortho)
sacroiliitis Ortho) / *inflammation of sacroiliac joint*
sacrospinalis (Ortho)
sacrum (Ortho) / *the section of vertebral column forming part of pelvis*
sagittal / *arrow straight / pertaining to a sagittal plane or direction*
SAH / subarachnoid hemorrhage
Sahli reaction / *converting hemoglobin into acid hematin with hydrochloric acid, and comparing color*
Saint Johnswort / St. John's wort / *herbal remedy*
Saint triad / *cholelithiasis, diverticulosis, hiatal hernia*
Sal-Acid plaster
salbutamol inhaler / albuterol / *bronchodilator* / D
Salflex / salsalate / *analgesic / antirheumatic / antipyretic* / D
salicylates / *antirheumatic / analgesic* / D
saline / *salty / pertaining to salt*
SalineX / sodium chloride / *nasal mist* / D [OTC]
salivary
salmeterol xinafoate / Serevent / *twice daily bronchodilator / for asthma* / D
Salmonella / *genus of bacteria*
salmonellosis / *infection with Salmonella bacteria*

Additional Entries

____

____

____

____

salon pain patch
salpingectomy (Gyn) / *surgical removal of a fallopian tube*
salpingo-oophoritis (Gyn) / *inflammation of an ovary*
salsalate / *analgesic / antipyretic / anti-inflammatory / anti-rheumatic* / D
saltatory / *proceeding by leaps*
Salutensin / Salutensin-Demi / *antihypertensive* / D
salvarsan / arsphenamine / D
Salzmann (Oph)
SAM / *systemic anterior motion*
sammoma...**NO!** / (see "psammoma")
Sampter syndrome
sanguineous / *blood*
Sansert / methysergide maleate / *for migraine and vascular head-aches* / D
SAO_2 / *arterial blood gas*
saphenous / *pertaining to a saphenous vein in leg / frequently used in coronary artery bypass graft surgery (CABG)*
sapr-, sapro- / *rot / rotten / putrid / decaying*
saprophyte/-ic / *living on decay*
sarc-, sarco- / *flesh*
Sarcoptes scabiei / *itch mite / mite that causes scabies in humans and mange in dogs*
Sarna / camphor, menthol and phenol / *cream for dry legs / counter-irritant* / D [OTC]
sat / saturation
satiety / *"elegant sufficiency"*
saturation
saucerized
SBE / subacute bacterial endocarditis / shortness (of) breath (on) exertion
scabiei / scabies

Additional Entries

---

scalene / *having sides of unequal length* / *pertaining to muscles*
scalenotomy / *surgery on anterior scalene muscle*
scalenus / *pertaining to scalene muscles*
scaler treadmill
scalp vein needle
scaly
scaphocephaly / *long, narrow skull*
scaphoid / *boat-shaped*
scapholunate
scapula/-ae (Ortho) / *shoulder blade*
scato- / feces
scatoma / stercoroma
Schamberg purpura (Derm) / *dermatitis in skin, ankles and feet of young males*
Schatzki ring
Schaumann sarcoid / S. sarcoidosis
Scheuermann disease (Ortho) / *osteochondrosis*
Schillings/B_{12} test / *for gastrointestinal absorption of vitamin B_{12}* / T
Schirmer test (Oph) / *for keratoconjuctivitis sicca* / T
schistocyte / *red blood corpusc*le
Schistosoma/-iasis / e.g., s. mansoni; s. japonicum; s. hematobium
schitz-, schitzo- / *split* / *divided*
schizophrenia (Psych) / *a mental disorder*
Schmidt syndrome / *paralysis on one side, affecting the vocal cord and trapezius* / *due to a lesion*
Schmorl nodule / *nodule seen in radiographs of the spine*
Schneider nail
schneiderian membrane / tunica mucosa nasi / *the nasal mucosa*
Schönlein-Henoch purpura / *nonthrombocytopenic purpura due to vasculitis*

Additional Entries

schwannoma / *benign neoplasm encapsulated in nerve sheath*

Schwartz test

sciatic / *pertaining to hip area* / e.g., s. nerve

sciatica / *radiating pain in back, hip or leg, usually due to herniated lumbar disk*

scintigraphy / *diagnostic procedure*

scintillation / *sparks*

scintigram / scintiscan

scintiphotography / *photographing scintillations emitted by radio-active substances injected into the body*

scirrhous CA / *hard cancer*

sclera- / *hard*

sclera (Oph) / *fibrous tissue forming outer envelope of the eye*

sclera nonicteric / *part of EENT physical examination*

scleral show

scleredema (Derm) / *nonpitting induration of the skin*

sclero- *hard*

sclerodactyly (Derm) / *localized scleroderma of the fingers*

scleroderma / *hardening and shrinking of connective tissue*

sclerodermatomyositis

sclerosis / *hardening*

sclerotherapy

scoliosis (Ortho) / *abnormal curvature of the spine*

-scop- / *look* / *observe* / *reveal*

scopolamine / *antispasmodic* / *anticholinergic* / D

-scopy / *an activity involving the use of an instrument for viewing*

scorbutic / *scurvy*

Scotch short arm (Ortho) / *leg cast*

scotoma / (pl.) scotomata (Oph) / *an area of lost vision within the visual field*

Scot-Tussin / *antitussive* / *antihistamine* / D

Additional Entries

---

scout film
screening urinalysis
Scribner shunt (Nephrology)
scrofula / *cervical tuberculous lymphadenitis / glandular swelling*
scybalum / *hard, dry stools*
Sea and Ski / *lotion*
sebaceous / *pertaining to glands that secrete oil / fat*
seborrheic keratoses
Sebulex / sulfur and salicylic acid / *shampoo*
sebum / *oily secretion of sebaceous glands*
Sebutone / *antiseborrheic / antipsoriatic / keratolytic /* D
Seconal / secobarbital / *sedative / hypnotic /* D
secondary to / *portrayed as "2°"*
secretory / *pertaining to secretion*
Sectral / acebutolol / *antihypertensive / antiarrhythmic /* D
secundines (Ob) / *afterbirth*
secundum artem / *professional manner*
sed rate / *sedimentation rate*
seg / *segmented neutrophils*
segmentation / *cleavage / division into smaller parts*
segmenters / *malarial organisms*
segs / *blood cells*
Seldane / *nonsedating antihistamine /* D
Seldinger technique / *in angiography*
selenium / *metallic element*
selenious
sella / saddle / e.g., s. turcica / *saddlelike bony prominence on upper part of the sphenoid bone*
Selsun / selenium sulfide / *cream / for tinea (fungal infection)*
SEM (Cardio) / scanning electron microscope

S

Additional Entries

semantic complaints

semen / *ejaculate of penis* / *fluid containing sperm* / *male seed*

semi- / *half* / *partially*

semimembranosus

seminiferous / *conveying semen*

seminoma / *tumor of the testis* / *germ cell tumor*

Semmes-Weinstein monofilament

Semprex-D / acrivastine and pseudoephedrine / *decongestant* / *antihistamine* / D

senescent/-cense / *old age* / *being old*

Senna Tabs / *laxative* / D [OTC]

Senokot / senna / *laxative* / D [OTC]

sensorineural

septi cavum pellucidi (Neuro) / *a triangular double membrane in the brain*

septic / *putrefactive* / *containing pus* / *pertaining to sepsis*

septoplasty / *surgical repair or correction of nasal septum*

Septra DS / co-trimoxazole / *anti-infective* / *antibacterial* / D

septum/septa / *wall* / *partition between two body cavities*

sequela / (pl.) sequelae / *condition following and resulting from a disease* / e.g., lesion caused by attack of disease

sequestrum / *piece of dead bone*

Ser-Ap-Es / hydralazine, hydrochlorothiazide and reserpine / *antihypertensive* / D

Serax / oxazepam / *anxiolytic* / D

Serentil / mesoridazine besylate / *antipsychotic* / D

Serevent inhaler / *bronchodilator for asthma* / D

sero- / *serum* / *serous*

serologies

seroma / *mass caused by accumulation of serum in tissue or organ*

seronegative / *absence of a specific antibody in serum*

Additional Entries

Serophene / clomiphene citrate / *ovulation stimulant* / D
seropurulent / *area containing serum and pus*
serosa / *outer layer of a visceral structure in body cavity*
serosanguineous / *pertaining to a discharge of serum and
    blood*
serositis / (pl.) serositides / *inflammation of a serous
    membrane*
serous otitis / *fluid in the ear canal*
serotonin / *vasoconstrictor*
Serpasil / *antihypertensive* / *antipsychotic* / D
serpiginous / *spreading*
Serratia / *bacteria*
Sertoli cell / *cells in columns* / e.g., S. cell tumor
Serzone / nefazodone / *antidepressant* / D
sesamoid / *resembling a sesame seed in size or shape* / e.g., s. bone
sessile / *attached widely at base, not pedunculated or like a stalk* /
    e.g., s. polyp
sestamibi / *new treadmill test* / T
seton procedure / *a thread or threads, strip of gauze, length of wire
    or other material passed through subcutaneous tissues as a
    guide for dilatation with larger instruments*
SGOT / serum glutamic oxaloacetic transaminase
SGPT /serum glutamic pyruvic transaminase
Sheldon catheter
shampoo, coal tar
shanker...**NO!** (see "chancre")
shave excisional / *in biopsy*
Sheehan syndrome / *hypopituitarism* / *caused by severe circulatory
    collapse postpartum*
Shenton line / *a curved line seen in x-ray of normal hip joint (top of
    obturator foramen)*

Additional Entries

Shieie syndrome / (pronounced "she-he") / *inherited metabolic disease*

Shigella / *microorganisms in enteritis*

Shiley tracheotomy tube

shingles / herpes zoster (Derm) / *blistering skin disease that affects peripheral nerves / caused by virus*

Shirodkar procedure encirclage (Gyn)) / *surgical placement of purse string suture around incompetent cervical os / to prevent premature onset of labor*

shock wave lithotripsy / *crushing of a stone in the bladder by means of shock waves*

short-colon exam / short colonoscopy

shotty nodes / *resemble buckshot*

SH renal disease

shunt/-ing / *bypass / divert / using mechanical means to divert accumulated fluids from body*

Shy-Drager syndrome / *chronic orthostatic hypotension*

sial-, sialo- / *saliva / salivary glands*

sialectasis/-ia / *dilation of a salivary duct*

sialoadenitis / sialadenitis / *inflammation of salivary glands*

sialogastrone / *substance in saliva*

sialogram / *x-ray of salivary ducts*

sialoaerophagy / *frequent swallowing, taking into the stomach abnormal quantities of saliva and air*

sibilant / *hissing*

sickle cell / *sickle- or crescent-shaped cells*

sicklemia / *having sickle- or crescent-shaped cells in blood*

sickle cell anemia

sider-, sidero- / *iron*

sideroachrestic process / *related to iron / anemia*

sideroblast / *iron in red blood cell*

Additional Entries

---

siderosis / *pneumoconiosis due to inhalation of iron particles*
sigmoid colon
sigmoidoscopy
signet ring cell
Sigvaris / *stockings*
sign, drawer
SI joint (Ortho) / sacroiliac
Silastic / *implant* / *trademark of silicone used in prostheses*
Silipos pad
Silvadene / silver sulfadiazine / cream / *for burns* / D
silver fork deformity / *in Colles fracture*
simethicone / *antiflatulent* / D [OTC]
Simmond disease / *panhypopituitarism*
simvastatin / Zocor / *antihyperlipidemic* / D
sinciput / *forehead and area just above it*
Sine-Aid / pseudoephedrine and ibuprofen / *decongestant* / *analgesic* / D [OTC]
Sinemet / levodopa and carbidopa / *antiparkinsonian* / D
Sinequan / doxepin / *anxiolytic* / *antidepressant* / D
singlet
singultus / *hiccups*
sinistro- / *left* / *toward the left*
sinistrocardia (Cardio) / *displacement of heart to the left*
sinistrocerebral (Neuro) / *pertaining to left cerebral hemisphere*
sinobronchial
sinus / (pl.) sinuses / *cavity* / *channel* / *hollow* / *channel for passage of blood or lymph*
sinus bradycardia (Cardio) / *abnormally slow heartbeat* / *originating in the normal sinus pacemaker*
sinusitis

Additional Entries

____

____

____

____

sinus trephination / *sawing a circular area with a trephine, for drainage*

sinus venosus (Cardio) / *in atrial septal defect* (ASD)

Sippy diet / *ulcer treatment*

sitz baths / *sitting in warm water* / *used to treat hemorrhoids*

Sjögren syndrome / *symptom complex of postmenopausal women*

Skelaxin / *skeletal muscle relaxant* / D

Skene gland (Gyn) / ductus para-urethrales urethrae femininae / *glands just inside of and on the posterior of urethra*

Skoal / *chewing tobacco*

SKSD / streptokinase streptodornase

SLE / systemic lupus erythematosus

sliding hiatal hernia

Slim Fast / *diet supplement*

Slinky balloon catheter

slit-lamp (Oph) / *eye exam*

Slo-bid / theophylline / *antiasthmatic* / *bronchodilator* / D

Slow-Mag / *magnesium supplement* / D

Slo-Niacin / niacin / *nutritional supplement* / D [OTC]

Slo-Phyllin / theophylline / *antiasthmatic* / *bronchodilator* / D

Slo-Phyllin GG / theophylline and guaifenesin / *antiasthmatic* / *bronchodilator* / *expectorant* / D

sloughing / (pronounced "sluff-ing") / *dead matter or necrosed tissue separated from living tissue*

Slow Fe / ferrous sulfate / *hematinic* / D [OTC]

Slow-K / potassium choride / *potassium supplement* / D

Sluder neuralgia

SMA-20 / Sequential Multiple Analysis (of 20 chemical constituents) / L

SMAC / Sequential Multiple Analyzer Computers / L

small bowel x-ray

Additional Entries

Small-Carrion penile prosthesis

Smith-Lemli-Opitz syndrome / *hereditary condition with multiple congenital anomalies*

smudging / *speech defect in which difficult consonants are omitted*

Snellen chart (Oph)

SNF / skilled nursing facility

snout reflex

snuffbox / *on making a fist, the triangular area formed by thumb and first finger / when snuff was used, a small pinch could be placed in this "box" and snuffed up into the nose*

SO / significant other

SO_4 / sulfate

soai...**NO!** (see "psoai")

soaked-cotton pledgets 4%

soas...**NO!** (see "psoas")

SOB / shortness of breath

sodium cellulose

Sodium Sulamyd (Oph) / *eye drops / ophthalmic bacteriostatic* / D

sodium valproate / Depakene / *anticonvulsant* / D

soft mechanical diet

soft-tissue mass

SOH / sympathetic orthostatic hypotension

Solaquin Forte / hydroquinone / *hyperpigmentation bleaching agent / sunscreen* / D

solar and actinic keratoses (Derm)

solar elastosis

soldier's heart (Cardio) / neurocirculatory asthenia

soleus muscle

Solu-Cortef / hydrocortisone / *glucocorticoids* / D

S

Additional Entries

____

____

____

____

Solu-Medrol / methylprednisolone / *glucocorticoid* / *anti-inflam-matory* / D
solute / *dissolved*
Soma / carisoprodol / *skeletal muscle relaxant* / D
somat-, somatico, somato- / *the body* / *pertaining to the body*
somatic / *pertaining to or affecting the body, as distinguished from a body part, the mind, or environment*
somatic complaints
somatization / *expressing psychological needs in physical symptoms*
somatoform
somatome
somatostatin / *growth hormone-release inhibiting factor* / D
somatotype / *type of human physique*
somn-, somni- / *sleep*
somnambulance / *sleepwalking*
somnolence/-ency / *sleepiness* / *inclination to sleep*
somnolent and obtunded
Somogyi units / S. effect / *amount of amylase to reduce to 1 mg. of glucose per 30 minutes*
sonogram / *display obtained by ultrasonic scanning*
soralen...**NO!** (see "Psoralen")
Sorbuthane / *shoe insert*
sorcon...**NO!** (see "Psorcon")
Soto syndrome / *cerebral gigantism*
souffle / *soft blowing sound*
Southern blot analysis / *DNA protein analysis*
SP / suprapubic
S/P / status post / e.g., his status is . . . having been hospitalized, having had pneumonia / *whatever past condition is being noted*
Sparine / promazine hydrochloride / *antipsychotic* / D
spasmodic / *of the nature of a spasm*

Additional Entries

spasm / *sudden involuntary contraction*
spasmus nutans (Neuro)
SPAT / slow paroxysmal atrial tachycardia
spear
Spectazole / econazole nitrate / *topical antifungal* / D
SPECT scan / single photon emission computerized
    tomography (scan)
Spenco metatarsal pad / *in shoes*
SPEP total protein/serum protein electrophoresis (total protein)
spermatocele / *cystic tumor containing spermatozoa*
spheno- / *wedge* / *wedge-shaped* / *the sphenoid bone*
sphenoid sinusitis
spherocytes / *spheroid-shaped erythrocytes observed in*
    hemolytic anemia
spherocytosis / *familial hemolytic anemia*
sphero- / *spherical* / *a sphere*
spherule / *small, spherical-shaped structure*
sphincter / *band of muscles encircling a body orifice*
sphincter of Oddi / *sheath of muscle fibers along bile and pancre-*
    atic passages
sphincterotomy
sphingolipidosis / *genetic metabolic disorders characterized by*
    neurological deterioration and blindness (amaurosis)
sphygmomanometer / *blood pressure cuff*
spica splint / *used for gamekeeper's thumb*
spicule / *small, needle-shaped body*
Spiegler-Fendt sarcoid / *lymphocytoma*
Spielmeyer-Vogt disease / *amaurotic idiocy* / *late juvenile cerebral*
    sphingolipidosis
spiff / dobutamine spiff (Cardio) / *three-day hospital treatment to*
    "spiff" up the heart

Additional Entries

---

spigelian line / *line on abdomen marking edge of rectus abdominis muscle*

spina bifida / *congenital defect in walls of spinal canal* / *lack of union between the laminae of vertebrae*

spina bifida occulta

spinatus

spina ventosa / *tuberculosis of the bone*

spine or CVAT / (spine or) costovertebral angle tenderness

spine of scapula

spinnbarkeit (Ob-Gyn) / *test for ovulation* / T

spinociliary reflex

spinous

spir-, spiro- / *coil* / *coil-shaped*

spiral reconstruction / *coiled or winding*

spirogram / *a tracing or graph of respiratory movements*

spirometer / *device used to measure respiratory gases*

spirometry (Pulm) / *gasometer for measuring respiratory gases*

spironolactone / *potassium-sparing diuretic* / *aldosterone antagonist* / D

Spirozide / hydrochlorothiazide and spironolactone (discontinued 1994) / *diuretic* / *antihypertensive* / D

spissated / inspissated / *thickened*

splanchn-, splanchni-, splanchno- / *viscera*

splanchnic / *pertaining to viscera*

splanchnolith / *an intestinal stone*

splanchnomicria / *smaller than normal splanchnic organs*

splen-, spleno- / *the spleen*

splenectomy / *excision of the spleen*

splenomegaly / *enlargement of the spleen*

splenosis / *growth of splenic tissue in abdomen*

spondyl-, spondylo- / *spinal column* / *vertebra*

Additional Entries

---

spondylolisthesis / *displacement of 5th lumbar vertebra*
spondylolysis / *dissolution of a vertebra*
spondylosis / *vertebral ankylosis* / e.g., s. cervical / *degener-
    ative arthritis* / *osteoarthritis of cervical vertebrae*
spondyloarthropathy / *disease of the joints of the spine*
spondylotomy / *incision of a vertebra* / *incision of the
    posterior arch of a vertebra* / *laminectomy*
spongioblastoma / *tumor containing embryonic epithelial
    cells*
spor-, spori-, sporo- / *seed* / *spore*
Sporanox / itraconazole / *systemic antifungal* / D
sporotrichosis / *fungus*
Sporotrichum schenchii / *a class of protozoa*
Sprengel deformity / *congenital elevation of the scapula*
sprue / *poor intestinal digestion and absorption with excessive
    excretion of fats in the feces (steatorrhea)*
    e.g., celiac s. / *celiac disease*
spun specimen
spur / *a projecting body, as from a bone*
squamous cell carcinoma
squamous dysplasia
SR (Cardio) / sinus rhythm
ST and T-wave, nonspecific / *electrocardiograph wave segments*
ST segment / *electrocardiograph wave segment*
stably
Stadol / butorphanol tartrate / *narcotic agonist-antagonist anal-
    gesic* / D
stage IV-A / *in Hodgkin disease*
staghorn calculus / *in kidney stone*
stainable iron
Stamm gastroplasty / *plastic operation on the stomach*

Additional Entries

____
____
____
____

stapedectomy (ENT) / *excision of the stapes (auditory ossicles)*
stapes (ENT) / *stirrup-shaped bone of ear*
staph / staphylococcus / *bacteria that cause serious opportunistic infections*
Staph aureus pneumonia
Staphylococcal aureus
Staphylococcus warneri
Staph epidermidis / *white colonies found on normal skin*
Staph hominis / *associated with infection of wounds*
startle test
stasis / *stoppage / stagnation*
STAT / L. *statum* / immediately
Statak sutures
Statham transducer / *transforms one form of energy to another*
stationary / *immobile*
status asthmaticus / *a particularly severe episode of asthma*
status post . . . / *patient's status is: post hospitalization, post pneumonia, or whatever past condition is being noted*
stear-, stearo-, steato- / *fat*
steatorrhea / *excretion of large amounts of fat in the feces, due to intestinal failure to digest and absorb it*
Steell murmur (Cardio) / *auscultatory cardiac sound*
Stein-Leventhal syndrome (Gyn) / *polycystic ovary disease*
Steinmann pin (Ortho) / *a metal rod for the internal fixation of fractures*
Stelazine / *antianxiety / antipsychotic / for schizophrenia* / D
stellate / *shaped like a star / rosette*
stellate laceration
stellate ganglion block / *for pain control*
steno- / *narrow / contracted / close / stricture*
stenosis/-es / *narrowing of any canal, especially cardiac valves*

Additional Entries

Stensen canal / *parotid duct*
stent / *mold* / *graft*
step 1 / *in low cholesterol diet*
stephanion (Neuro) / *part of skull*
sterco- / *feces*
stercoraceous / *relating to feces* / *containing feces*
stereognosis / *knowing by sense of touch*
stereotactic / stereotaxic / *in brain surgery* / *in brain biopsy*
Sterile H$_2$O for injection
Sterile NaCl / *saline*
Steri-Strips
sterile / *aseptic, free of microorganisms and their spores* /
    inability to fertilize or reproduce
sterilely
stern-, sterno- / *the sternum* / *pertaining to the sternum*
sternal heart border
Sternberg-Reed cells / Sternberg's giant cells
sternocleidomastoid / *pertaining to the sternum, clavicle, and*
    mastoid process
sternomanubrial
stenosis/-tic / *narrowed*
sternotomy / *cutting through the sternum*
stertorous breathing / *snoring* / *noisy breathing during sleep*
stethoscope
Stevens-Johnson syndrome / *sometimes fatal erythema multiforme,*
    with flulike beginning, then severe mucocutaneous lesions
sthen-, stheno- / *strength and activity*
sthenia / *a condition of strength and excessive vital force*
sthenic / *sturdy* / *strongly built*
sthenic habitus / *active, strong body*
stigma / (pl.) stigmata

Additional Entries

Still's disease

stillbirth / *birth of an infant who died prior to delivery* / *dead fetus*

stillborn / *born dead* / *an infant dead at birth*

St. John's wort / Saint Johnswort / *herbal remedy*

stocking distribution / glove distribution / *sensation going up the extremity evenly on both sides, as when putting on stockings or gloves*

stom-, stomat-, stomato- / *mouth*

stoma/-s/-ata / *artificial opening between two cavities or canals* / *a tiny opening or pore*

stomatitis / *inflammation of the mouth's mucous membrane*

stomatocytes / *a form of red blood cell as seen in hemolytic anemia and in liver disease*

stomocephalus / *deformed fetus with very small head and neck*

stool color / *yellow-brown = yellow **to** brown* / *yellow/brown = yellow **and** brown*

strabismus (Oph) / *squinting*

strangury / *slow urine*

stratum / strata / *layer*

strep / Streptococcus / agalacticae

strep faecium

strept-, strepto- / *twist*

streptococcus agalactia / *found in raw milk* / *associated with human infections, especially of infants*

streptococcus bovis (and mitis) / *found in the alimentary tract of cattle and sometimes in human feces*

streptodornase / *a deoxyribonuclease produced by hemolytic streptococci*

streptokinase / *a protein that binds plasminogen* / *used in clot removal*

streptomycin / *aminoglycoside* / *bactericidal antibiotic* / *primary tuberculostatic* / D

Addditional Entries

---

streptozocin / streptozotocin / Zanosar / *antibiotic anti-neoplastic* / D

streptozyme test / T

Stresstabs / *vitamin supplement* / D

striae / *narrow bands* / *stretch marks*

stridor / *harsh respiration*

stroke / *brain damage caused by leaking blood vessels or interruption of blood supply*

strom/-ata / *framework, usually of connective tissue*

stromal / stromic

Strongyloides stercolaris

strut / *support*

Stryker collar

S

STT-wave changes (Cardio) / *electrocardiograph wave segment*

Stuart factor / thrombokinase / *pertaining to coagulation*

Stuartinic / *hematinic* / D

styloid / *long, pointed*

Stypven / *viper venom* / T

sub- / *under* / *almost* / *less than normal* / *inferior*

sub.q. q.a.m. / subcutaneous, every morning

subacromial / *under the acromion process*

subarachnoid (Neuro) / *beneath the arachnoid membrane*

subastragalar (Ortho) / *beneath the calcaneus*

subcarinal / *beneath a ridgelike structure*

subchondral / *beneath or below rib cartilages*

subclavian / *beneath the clavicle* / e.g., s. artery; s. vein

subclavian / Quinton / *catheter*

subcostal / *beneath rib or ribs* / *certain arteries, veins, nerves*

subendocardial (Cardio)

sublimis / *near the surface* / e.g., s. tendon / *superficial t.*

sublingual / *beneath the tongue*

Additional Entries

---

subluxation / *incomplete dislocation*
submandibular
submental nodes / *below the chin*
subnasal
subpapillary / *eruption of a few or scattered papules*
subpial (Neuro) / *beneath pia*
subserous / subserosal / *beneath serous membrane*
substernal
subtalar arthritis / *arthritis inferior to the talus/foot*
subtilisin / *proteolytic enzyme isolated from soil bacteria, which catalyzes peptide bonds*
subtract serial sevens
subungual / *beneath a nail* / *hyponychial*
subxiphoid
succedaneum / *substitute for a drug or therapeutic agent*
succussed / *moving fluid*
sucrose lysis test
Sudafed / pseudoephedrine / *nasal decongestant* / D [OTC]
Sudephedrine...**NO!** (see "pseudoephedrine")
Sudeck atrophy / *post-traumatic osteoporosis*
sudor- / *sweat* / *perspiration*
sudoresis / *profuse sweating*
sugar tong splint
sui generis / *unique* / *of its particular kind* / *forming a kind by itself*
Sulamyd / Sodium Sulamyd / *eye drops* / *ophthalmic bacteriostatic* /D
Sular / nisoldipine / *antihypertensive* / *calcium channel blocker* / D
sulcus/-sulci / *groove*
sulfacetamide / *bacteriostatic antibiotic* / D
Sulfamethoprim / trimethoprim / *anti-infective* / D
sulfamethoxazole/ *broad-spectrum antibiotic* / D
sulfasalazine / *broad-spectrum bacteriostatic* / D

Additional Entries

____
____
____
____

sulfhydryl group
sulfisoxazole / *broad-spectrum bacteriostatic* / D
sulfonamide
sulfonylurea assay / T
sulindac / *nonsteroidal anti-inflammatory* / *for arthritis* / D
sumatriptan / *antimigraine* / D
Sumycin / tetracycline / *broad-spectrum antibiotic* / D
super- / *above* / *excess*
superciliary / *eyebrow*
super-fatted soap
superior axis
supernumerary / *greater than the normal number*
supervene/-vening / *a condition occurring in addition to an already existing one*
supine/-ated / *lying on the back*
suppurative / *forming pus* / *containing pus*
supra- / *above* / *over*
supraclavicular / *above the clavicle*
supracondylar / *superior to a condyle*
supranuclear palsy / *occurring on the surface of a nucleus in the nervous system*
suprapatellar, bursa / *a bursa between the distal end of the femur and the quadriceps tendon*
suprapubic / *superior to the pubic arch*
suprasellar
supraspinatus / *muscle*
suprasternal notch / *superior to the sternum*
supravital / *staining method*
Suprax / cefixime / *cephalosporin-type antibiotic* / D
sura / sural / *pertaining to the calf of the leg*
sural nerve conduction / *pertaining to the calf of the leg*

S

Additional Entries

Surfak / docusate / *stool softener* / D [OTC]
Surmontil / trimipramine maleate / *tricyclic antidepressant* / D
Sustacal / *diet supplement* / *enteral nutritional therapy*
sustained release / *continuous acting* / D
Sustaire / theophylline / *timed-release bronchodilator* / *for asthma* / D
sustentaculum tali / *a process of the calcaneus which supports the talus*
suture / *a form of fibrous joint in which two bones are united by a fibrous membrane* / *to unite two surfaces by stitching* / *a seam, either natural or surgical* / *the material with which two surfaces are kept in apposition* / e.g., chromic catgut; Vicryl
SVT / supraventricular tachycardia
Swan-Ganz catheter / *soft catheter with balloon at the tip* / *for measuring pulmonary arterial pressures*
swimmer's view / *x-ray*
sycosis...**NO!** (see "psychosis")
syllium...**NO!** (see "psyllium")
Sylvian / *fissure*
Symadine / amantadine / *antiviral* / *antiparkinsonian agent* / D
Syme amputation / *amputation of the foot at the ankle joint*
Symmetrel / amantadine / *antiviral* / *antiparkinsonian agent* / D
sympath-, sympatheto-, sympathico, sympatho- / *the sympathetic part of the autonomic nervous system*
sympathectomy / *surgical removal of sympathetic nerve*
sympathomimetics / *adrenergic* / *mimicking effects of impulses in the sympathetic nervous system*
symphysis / *growing together*
symphysis pubis / *the joint formed by pubic bones of fibrocartilage* / *bony eminence under the pubic hair*
symptomatology / *the science of disease symptoms*
syn- / *union* / *association* / *together*

Additional Entries

Synalar-HP/fluocinolone acetonide/ *topical corticosteroid/*D **S**

Synalar solution / fluocinolone acetonide / *topical cortico-steroid* / D

Synalgos-HP / *narcotic analgesic* / D

Synarel / nafarelin acetate/*gonadotropin-releasing hormone/ for endometriosis* / D

synarthrosis/-es / *pertaining to joints*

synchondrosis/-es (Ortho)

syncope (pronounced "sync-o-pee") / *to swoon* / *to faint*

syncytium/-ia/-tial / *a protoplasmic mass*

syndactyly / *anomaly* / *hands*

syndesm-, syndesmo- / *ligament* / *ligamentous*

syndesmophyte / *bony growth on ligament*

syndesmosis / *type of fibrous joint*

synechia / *adhesion*

synophrys / *eyebrows growing together*

synostosis / bony ankylosis (Ortho) / *osseous union between bones forming a joint*

synovia/-ial / *lubricating fluid secreted by certain membranes, as those of joints*

synovioma / *synovial tumor involving a joint or tendon sheath*

synovitis / *inflammation of synovial membrane*

Synthroid / levothyroxine / *thyroid hormone* / D

syphilis / *sexually transmitted disease*

syringomyelia / *presence of abnormal tissue in spinal cord*

syrinx / *fistula* / *tube* / *pipe*

systole / (pronouned "syst-o-lee")

systolic / *top blood pressure number*

systolic ejection murmur (Cardio) / *cardiac murmur* / *due to regurgitation*

Additional Entries

____

____

____

____

T1—T12 / *first to twelfth thoracic vertebrae or nerves*
T7, T8 / "T7 to 8"
T&A / tonsillectomy and adenoidectomy
tabes dorsalis / *wasting*
Tac / *triamcinolone acetonide cream*
tachistoscope / *a device that projects a series of images onto a screen at rapid speed to test visual perception, memory and learning*
tachy- / *fast* / *rapid*
tachyarrhythmia (Cardio)
tachypnea/-neic / *rapid breathing*
TAF / *machine*
tacrine / Cognex / *Alzheimer treatment* / *cognition adjuvant for Alzheimer dementia* / D
tactile / *pertaining to touch or sense of touch* / e.g., t. fremitus
Taekwondo / *type of martial art*
Taenia / *tapeworm*
Tagamet / *gastric and duodenal ulcer treatment* / D
TAH (Gyn) / total abdominal hysterectomy
Tai Chi / *type of martial art*
Talacen / pentazocine compound / *narcotic agonist-antagonist* / *analgesic* / *antipyretic* / D
talar navicular / talonavicular joint (Ortho) / *ankle-foot area*
talc poudrage / *application of powder to a surface to promote fusion*
talipes / *any deformity of the foot involving the talus (ankle bone)* / e.g., t. equinus
talipedic / *clubfooted*
talocrural / *leg*
talus / (pl.) tali / *ankle* / *ankle bone*
Talwin / *narcotic agonist-antagonist analgesic* / D
Tambocor / flecainide / *antiarrhythmic* / D

Additional Entries

____

____

____

____

tambour / *sound*
tamoxifen / Nolvadex (Chemo)/ *for metastasized breast cancer* / D
tamponade / tamponage (Cardio) / *insertion of a tampon*
tandem ICON / *brand name of a pregnancy test* / T
Tanner stave V
Tapazole / methimazole / *antithyroid agent* / D
tardive / *late, especially when characteristic sign or symptom appears late in the course of the disease*
Tarlov cyst / *perineurial cyst* / *layer of connective tissue in a peripheral nerve*
tarso- / *edge of eyelid*
tarsometatarsal / *pertaining to foot and ankle bones*
tarsorrhaphy (Oph)
tarsotomy (Oph)
taurine / "low-taurine diet" / *sulfur-containing amine occurring in the bile*
Tavist-1 / *antihistamine* / D [OTC]
Tavist-D / *decongestant* / *antihistamine* / D
-taxon / *order* / *phylum*
Tay-Sachs disease / *fatal hereditary disease of children, found primarily in Jewish populations*
taxis / *manual replacement or reduction of a hernia or dislocation*
TB / tuberculosis
TBE / tick-borne encephalitis
TBG / thyroid binding globulin
TBI / thyroid binding index
Td booster / Tetanus and diphtheria (booster)
teaspoonfuls
technetium / *artificial radioactive element*
tectum/-a / *roof* / *roofed structure* / e.g., t. mesencephali (Neuro)
TED hose / *used in thromboembolic disease*

Additional Entries

Tedral / theophylline, ephedrine, and phenobarbital / *anti-asthmatic / bronchodilator / decongestant / sedative* / D

TEE / transesophageal echocardiography

Tegaderm / D

Tegison / etretinate / *systemic antipsoriatic* / D

tegmen / *a structure that covers*

Tegopen / cloxacillin sodium / *bactericidal antibiotic* / D

Tegretol / carbamazepine / *anticonvulsant* / D

teichoic acid / *polymers in gram-positive bacteria*

telagia / *referred pain / pain felt at a distance from its stimulus*

telangiectasia/-tatic / *procedure involving dilation of blood vessels / dilation of small or terminal blood vessels*

telemetry / *measuring body signals and transmitting results by radio signal to a distant location where data is reviewed and documented* / e.g., cardiac t. / *transmission of heart signals to a monitoring station*

teleroentgenogram / teleradiography / *x-ray radiography*

Telfa dressing

telogen / *resting phase of hair growth cycle*

temafloxacin / *antibacterial* / D

temazepam / *minor tranquilizer / hypnotic* / D

Tembid / *sustained action capsule* / D

Temovate Cream / clobetasol dipropionate / *topical corticosteroid / anti-inflammatory* / D

temp / *temperature*

temporo- / *temporal / temple*

temporomandibular / *pertaining to the temporal bone and the mandible*

ten(10)-EDAM

tenacious / *holding fast / persistent / stubborn / viscous / sticky*

Additional Entries

Tenckhoff catheter
tendinitis / tendonitis / *inflammation of a tendon*
   e.g., Achilles t. / t. calcaneus / *tendinitis of heel tendon*
tendo Achillis / Achilles tendon
tenesmus / *ineffectual straining*
Tenex / guanfacine / *antihypertensive / antiadrenergic* / D
teno- / *tendon*
tenoid...**NO!** (see"ctenoid")
Tenoretic / atenolol and chlorthalidone / *antihypertensive* / D
Tenormin / atenolol / *antianginal / antihypertensive / beta blocker* /D
tenosynovitis / *tendon sheath inflammation*
TENS unit (Ortho) / *electrical stimulation*
Tensilon test (Oph) / T
tensor / *any muscle that makes a part tense*
Tenuate Dospan / diethylpropion / *anorexiant* / D
teratogen / *causes birth defects*
teratoma / *ovary or testis growth*
Terazol / terconazole / *vaginal suppositories / antifungal* / D
terazosin / Hytrin / *antihypertensive* / D
terbutaline inhaler / *bronchodilator* / D
terion...**NO!** / (see "pterion")
Terramycin / *tetracycline-type antibiotic* / D
terrazzo / *tile floor*
Terry nail / *associated with liver disease, especially cirrhosis*
tertiary / third / *following "primary" and "secondary"*
terygium...**NO!** (see "pterygium")
Teslac / testolactone / *adjunctive hormonal chemotherapy / for*
   advanced postmenopausal breast carcinoma / D
Tessalon Perles / benzonatate / *antitussive* / D
testalgia / *pain in the testes, often a symptom in prostatitis*
testicular / *pertaining to the testes*

Additional Entries

Testoderm patch / *for scrotal area* / *hormone replacement therapy* / *for hypogonadism* / T

testosterone patch / *for age-related hormone deficiencies* / *no effect on prostate gland* / D

testosterone / *prolactin*

tetan-, tetano- / *tetanus* / *tetany*

tetanus / *disease caused by a neurotropic toxin*

tetany / *neurological syndrome characterized by twitching, cramps, spasms, and seizures*

tetra- / *four*

tetracetate / *preservative used in medicines*

tetracycline / *bacteriostatic antibiotic* / *antirickettsial* / D

tetralogy of Fallot (Cardio) / *four defects in the heart*

Tetrameres / *worms*

thalamic (Neuro) / *pertaining to the thalamus, part of the brain*

TFT / thyroid function test

thalassemia / *inherited disorder of hemoglobin metabolism* / e.g., t. intermedia

Thalitone / *antihypertensive* / *diuretic* / D

thallium / *diagnostic radioactive isotope*

Thayer-Martin / *GC culture* / *gonococcus culture*

thecoma (Gyn) / *type of neoplasm*

Theelin injections (discontinued 1995) / *estrogen replacement therapy* / *antineoplastic* / *for prostatic cancer* / *for breast cancer* / D

thelarche / *development of breasts at puberty*

thenar eminence / *the mound on the palm at the base of the thumb*

Theo-Dur / theophylline / *bronchodilator* / D

Theochron / *bronchodilator* / D

Theolair / theophylline / *antiasthmatic* / D

theophylline / *antiasthmatic* / D

Additional Entries

Theo-24 / *bronchodilator* / D
Thera-Band exercises
Theragran / *vitamin supplement* / D
thermophore / *apparatus for retaining heat* / *used in therapeutic local application*
thiamine HC / *salt of thiamine* / *for thiamine deficiency state*
thiabendazole / Mintezol / *anthelmintic* / *for worms* / D
thiazides / *diuretics*
thick and thin prep
Thiersch graft / *skin grafting method* / *used in transplantation*
thimerosal / *solution*
thioguanine / *antimetabolic antineoplastic* / D
thioridazine / Mellaril
thiotepa / *alkylating antineoplastic* / D
thiothixene / Navane / *antipsychotic* / D
thiourea / *treatment for Graves disease*
thorac-, thoracico-, thoraco- / *thorax* / *the chest*
thoracentesis / pleuracentesis / *surgical puncture of the chest wall for aspiration of fluids*
thoracic outlet syndrome / TOS / *compromised blood vessels or nerve fibers between base of neck and axilla*
thoracolumbar / *pertaining to thoracic and lumbar parts of spine*
thoracoscopy / *diagnostic examination of the chest (the pleural cavity) with an endoscope*
thoracotomy / *surgical incision of the wall of the chest*
Thorazine / chlorpromazine / *tranquilizer* / *antiemetic* / D
THR / total hip replacement
thromb-, thrombo- / *blood clot* / *blood coagulation*
thrombosed hemorrhoids
thrombocythemia / thrombocytosis / *abnormal increase of platelets in the blood*

Additional Entries

---

thrombocytopenia / thrombopenia / *abnormally small number of platelets in the blood*

thromboembolism / *embolism (obstruction) from a thrombus (clot)*

thromboembolic disease

thromboplastin / *a substance having procoagulant properties or activity*

thrombus / *clot in the cardiovascular system*

thym-, thymi-, thymo- / *the thymus / mind or emotions / wartlike*

thymectomy

thymoma

thyr-, thyro- / *the thyroid gland*

thyroglobulin / *glycoprotein occurring in the thyroid gland*

thyroglossal / *pertaining to the thyroid gland and the tongue*

thyroid function studies / TFTs

Thyrolar-2 / *thyroid hormone therapy* / D

thyromegaly / *thyroid enlargement*

thyroxine / free thyroxine index / *thyroxine is used in treatment of hypothyroidism*

TIA / transient ischemic attack

Tiazac / diltiazem / *antihypertensive / antianginal / calcium channel blocker* / D

TIBC / total iron binding capacity / T

tibia (Ortho) / *shin bone*

tibial arteries

tibial tuberosities

tic douloureux

-tic / *pertaining to words ending in -**sis*** / e.g., eme**sis**; eme**tic**

Ticlid / ticlopidine / *platelet aggregation inhibitor / for stroke* / D

ticlopidine HCl / Ticlid / D

Additional Entries

____

____

____

____

t.i.d. / L. *ter in die* / three times a day
Tietze syndrome / *painful swelling of second rib* / *may mimic coronary artery disease*
Tigan / trimethobenzamide / *suppositories* / *antiemetic* / D
Tilade / nedocromil sodium / *antiasthmatic* / D
TILS / tumor-infiltrating lymphocytes
tilt table testing / T
Timentin / ticarcillin and clavulanic acid / *penicillin-type antibiotic*/D
Timolide / *antihypertensive* / D
timolol / *atenolol* / *antiadrenergic* / D
Timoptic / timolol / *topical antiglaucoma agent* / D
Tinactin cream / tolnaftate / *topical antifungal* / D [OTC]
tinctorial / *staining*
tinea / *a fungus infection*
    t. corporis / *"ringworm of the body"*
    t. cruris / *in male groin*
    t. faciei / *of the face (other than bearded area)*
    t. manus / *of the hands*
    t. pedis / *athlete's foot*
    t. unguium / *"ringworm of the nail"*
    t. versicolor / *fungus* / *depigmented rash* / *multiple macular patches*
Tinel sign / *tingling on percussion*
tinnitus (Oto) / *ringing in the ears* / *noises in the ears*
Tinver lotion / sodium thiosulfate / *topical antifungal* / D
TIP / terminal interphalangeal
tires / *condition marked by constipation, vomiting, tremors, pain*
tiring (Ortho) / *fastening wire around fragments of a bone*
tirofiban / Aggrastat / *prevents blood clot formation* / D
Tiselius apparatus / *to separate proteins of blood serum, plasma and other body fluids by electrophoresis*

Additional Entries

tissue plasminogen activator, recominant / t-PA / TPA /
   dissolves blood clots / D
titer / *standard of strength of a volumetric test solution* /
   quantity of a substance required to produce reaction
   with a given volume of another substance
Titralac Plus Liquid / *antacid* / *antiflatulent* / D [OTC]
titrate / *to determine given component in solution by adding*
   liquid reagent of known strength until changes in color
titubation / *staggering* / *reeling*
Tizac...**NO!** (see "Tiazac") / D
TKR / total knee replacement
TM / tympanic membrane
TMJ / temporomandibular joint
TNTC / too numerous to count
tobaccoism
tobramycin / *antibacterial antibiotic* / D
Tobrex / tobramycin (Oph) / *ophthalmic antibiotic* / D
tocolytics (Ob-Gyn) / *drugs to stop labor*
Tofranil / imipramine / *tricyclic antidepressant* / D
tolazamide / *antidiabetic* / D
tolbutamide / *antidiabetic* / D
Tolectin DS / tolmetin sodium / *nonsteroidal anti-inflammatory* / D
Tolinase / tolazamide / *antidiabetic* / D
tolnaftate / *cream* / *antifungal* / D
-tome / *cutting instrument*
tomograms
tono- / *tone* / *tension*
tonoclonic / *twitching*
Tonocard / tocainide / *antiarrhythmic* / D
tonsil / *any group of lymphoid tissue* / e.g., cerebellar t.;
   eustacian t; lingual t.; palatine t.; pharyngeal t.

Additional Entries

tonsillar / tonsillitis

tonsillectomy

tonsillopharyngitis

tophaceous / *gritty*

tophus / *gout* / *chalky deposit*

Topicort gel / *topical corticosteroidal anti-inflammatory* / D

Toprol XL / desoxymethasone / *antihypertensive* / *long-term antianginal* / *beta blocker* / D

Toradol injection / ketorolac tromethamine / *analgesic* / *nonsteroidal anti-inflammatory* / *for acute, moderately severe pain* / D

torcular Herophili / *confluence of sinuses*

tori palatinus

Torecan / thiethylperazine maleate / *antiemetic* / D

tormina / *colic*

Tornalate / bitolterol mesylate / *bronchodilator* / D

torsades de pointes (Cardio)

torsemide / Demadex / *loop diuretic* / D

torticollis / *neck* / *contracted muscle*

tortuous / *many curves, turns or twists*

tortuosity

torulus (Derm) / *a small elevation* / *a papilla*

Torulopsis glabrata

torulosis / cryptococcosis / *an infection with a predilection for the brain and meninges* / *invades the central nervous system (CNS) and is fatal if left untreated*

torus / *throat* / *palate*

TOS / thoracic outlet syndrome

tosis...**NO!** (see "ptosis")

Tourette syndrome

tox-, toxi-, toxico, toxo- / *poison*

toxignomic / *having toxic action peculiar to a poison*

Additional Entries

____

____

____

____

Toxoplasma/-plasmosis / *protozoa comprising parasites of many organs and tissues of birds and mammals, including humans*

t-PA / TPA / alteplase, recombinant / *tissue plasminogen activator / blood clot dissolver* / D

TPR / temp, pulse (and) respiration

T&R / tenderness and rebound

trabecula/-ae / *supporting bundle of tissue fibers / small piece of spongy bone*

trabeculation / *trabecula on the walls of an organ or body part / the process of forming spongy bone*

trace ankle edema

trace occult blood / *hidden blood in the stool*

trace positive

trache-, trachel-, trachelo- / *neck*

trachea/-eal / *air tube from the larynx into the thorax*

tracheitis

tracheobronchitis

tragus (ENT) / *cartilaginous projection on ear*

Trancopal / *anxiolytic* / D

Trandate / labetalol / *antihypertensive* / D

trandolapril / Mavik / *antihypertensive / ACE inhibitor* / D

trans- / *through / across / beyond*

transaminases / amidinotransferases / *enzymes*

Transderm Scopolamine / Transderm Scop

transducer / *device that converts energy from one form to another*

transesophageal echocardiogram (TEE) / *fiberoptic endoscope into esophagus for two-dimensional images or Doppler information*

transferase / *an enzyme*

transferrin / *a globulin in plasma*

transient / *brief / short-lived* / e.g., t. global amnesia

Additional Entries

____

____

____

____

transilluminate / transilluminal / *passing light through tissues or a body cavity*

transsphenoidal / *through or across the sphenoid bone*

transudate / *fluid that has passed through membrane or extruded from blood as a result of hydrodynamic forces*

transurethral / *through the urethra*

Trans-Ver-Sal / salicylic acid / *transdermal patch / topical keratolytic* / D

Tranxene / clorazepate dipotassium / *anxiolytic* / D

trapeze

trapezius / trapezii

Traube space / *part of the thorax over which the air in the stomach produces a tympanic sound*

traumatopnea / *passage of air in and out of a wound in chest wall*

trazodone / Desyrel / *antidepressant* / D

treadmill, scaler

treadmill, thallium

treadmill, sestamibi

Treitz arch / *artery and vein form arch between duodenum and left kidney*

Trental / pentoxifylline / *hemorheologic agent / to improve blood microcirculation* / D

Trendelenburg position / *head of bed down 30-40º, and bed angulated beneath the knees*

trephination / *surgical procedure on cranium using a trephine*

trephine / *saw used for removal of a disc of bone from skull*

Treponema / *bacteria*

trepopnea / *condition in which breathing is most comfortable with patient turned in recumbent position*

tretinoin gel / Retin-A / *keratolytic / acute leukemia treatment* / D

tri- / three

Additional Entries

T_3RIA / *thyroid test* / T

triaditis / *inflammation of three elements considered as a unit*

triamcinolone acetonide / *corticosteroid* / *inhalant for asthma* / D

Triaminic / *decongestant* / *antihistamine* / *for allergy* / D

triamterene / Dyrenium / *potassium-sparing diuretic* / D

Triavil / amitriptyline and perphenazine / *antipsychotic* / *antidepressant* / D

tribade / *a lesbian*

Trichinella / *nematode parasite*

trichloroacetaldehyde / *chloral*

trich-, trichi-, tricho- / *hair* / *condition of hair*

trichalgia / *pain caused by touching the hair*

trichiasis / *hair that causes discomfort by turning inward into a body orifice* / e.g., inverted eyelashes

trichinosis / *disease caused by eating raw or near-raw pork that contains the nematode parasite Trichinella spiralis*

trichobezoar / *hair ball*

Trichocephalus / *nematode*

trichomonads / Trichomonadidae / *protozoan flagellates*

Trichomonas hominis / *protozoan flagellate*

trichomoniasis / *infection with trichomonas*

trichophytin / *culture*

trichophyton / rubrum / *fungus*

trichotillomania / *compulsion to pull out one's own hair*

trichuriasis / *infection with nematodes of genus Trichuria*

Trichuris / *intestinal parasite*

Tri-Cyclen / *birth control* / D

Tridesilon Creme / desonide / *topical corticosteroid anti-inflammatory* / D

Additional Entries

____

____

____

____

trifid / *split into three parts*
trifluoperazine / Stelazine / *antipsychotic* / *sedative* / D
trigeminal / *pertaining to the fifth cranial or trigeminus nerve*
trigeminy / trigeminal rhythm
triglycerides / *fatty substances in the blood*
trigonitis (Uro) / *inflammation of the bladder*
triiodothyronine / *radioactive agent*
Trilafon / *antipsychotic* / *antidopaminergic* / *antiemetic* / D
Tri-Levlen / ethinyl estradiol and levonorgestrel / *triphasil oral contraceptive* / D
Trilisate / choline magnesium trisalicylate / *analgesic* / *antipyretic* / *anti-inflammatory* / D
trimeclizine / D
trimethoprim / sulfamethoxazole DS / *antibacterial antibiotic* / D
Trimox / amoxicillin / *penicillin-type antibiotic* / D
Trimpex / trimethoprim / *anti-infective* / *antibacterial* / D
Trinalin / azatadine and pseudoephedrine / *inhalation aerosol* / *decongestant* / *antihistamine* / D
Trinicon / D
Tri-Norinyl / ethinyl estradiol and norethindrone / *oral contraceptive* / D
Trinsicon / *hematinic* / D
triolein - T^{131}
trip- / *rub* / *friction* / also, **tripsy-** / *crushing*
Triphasil / *triphasic oral contraceptive* / D
triquetrum / *three-cornered*
trismus / *lockjaw* / *tetanus*
trisomy / *a cell or a person with an extra chromosome*
Tritec / ranitidine bismuth citrate / *histamine H^2 agonist for duodenal ulcers with H. pylori infection* / D
trochanter (Ortho) / *bony prominence in upper femur*

Additional Entries

trochanter roll / *roll placed against hip to maintain position*

trochanteric (Ortho) / *either of two processes below neck of femur*

troches / *medicated lozenges for mouth or throat*

trochlea / *a body structure that works as a pulley*

troglitazone Sankyo study / *antidiabetic* / D

-trophic / *nutrition*

-trophy / *development* / *growth* / e.g., hyper**trophy** / *over-development;* **atrophy** / *without growth*

trough of dosage / *in the morning*

Trousseau phenomenon / *spasmodic contractions of muscles upon pressure of nerves which go to them*

TRP / tubular reabsorption phosphate

truncal / *pertaining to trunk of body*

Trusopt (Oph) / *eye drops* / *topical carbonic anhydrase inhibitor* / *for glaucoma*

trypanosome / *genus of flagellate protozoa*

Trypanosoma / e.g., t. cruzi; t. gambiense

trypanosomiasis / *any disease caused by a trypanosome*

trypsinogen / *the inactive proenzyme of trypsin secreted by the pancreas*

TSH / thyroid stimulating hormone

tubercle / *small, rounded lesion* / *produced by infection with Myco-bacterium tuberculosis*

tuberculous / *affected with tuberculosis*

tuberosity / *an elevation* / *a protuberance*

tubotympanic/-al (Oto) / *pertaining to the eustachian tube and the tympanic cavity of the ear*

tubotympanitis (Oto)

tubular / villous adenoma / *adenomatous polyp of the colon whose cells are arranged in tubules*

Additional Entries

---

tubular reabsorption

Tuinal / amobarbital and secobarbital / *sedative* / *hypnotic* / D

tularemia / *disease transmitted to humans from rodents*

tularensis agglutinins / tularemia / deer fly fever / rabbit fever /
acute, plaguelike infectious disease / *caused by Francisella
tularensis* / *transmitted by direct contact with infected animals* /
named for Tulare, California, where disease was first discovered

TULIP study / *procedure for benign prostatic hyperplasia*

Tulis heel cushion

tumefaction / *swelling* / *edema*

tumorigenesis/-ic / *producing new tumor growth(s)*

tunica albuginea / *dense white collagenous covering around a
structure*

TUR / transurethral resection

turbinate/-s (Ortho) / *shaped like a top*

turgor / *swollen* / *congested*

Turner mosaic / *in a cell culture, two cell lines that are genotypically
distinct, but are derived from a single zygote*

Turner syndrome / *gonadal dysgenesis* / *absence of the second sex
chromosome*

TURP / transurethral resection (of) prostate

Tuss-Delay / D

Tussionex / hydrocodone and chlorpheniramine / *narcotic antitussive* /
antihistamine / D

Tussi-Organidin / *for cough* / D

Tuss-Ornade / *antitussive* / *decongestant* / D

TWAR titer / *form of Chlamydia that causes pneumonia*

tylectomy / *surgical removal of swelling or tumor*

tyloma / *callus*

Tylox / oxycodone and acetaminophen / *narcotic analgesic* /D

tympanic (Oto) / *resonant* / *pertaining to the tympanum*

Additional Entries

____

____

____

____

tympanitic membranes
tympanitis (Oto) / otitis media / *inflammation of the middle ear*
tympanogram (Oto)
tympanum (Oto) / *eardrum / the tympanic cavity / the middle ear*
tyramine / *for headaches*
tyzanidine / *experimental drug* / D
Tzanck / *cell test* / T

T

UA / urinalysis
UGI / UGIT / upper gastrointestinal (tract)
UGIS / upper gastrointestinal series
-ular / *relating to* / *resembling* / e.g., cir**cular**; valv**ular**
-ulation / *act of* / e.g., encaps**ulation**
-ule / *little globule* / e.g., caps**ule**
ulna (Ortho) / *forearm* / *side opposite of thumb*
ulnar gutter splint (Ortho) / *designed to restrict or correct ulnar deviation*
ulnocarpal joint
Ultralente / Insulin / D
Ultram / *analgesic* / D
Ultrase / *digestive enzymes* / *for pancreatic insufficiency* / D
ultrasonography / *echoes of pulses of ultrasonic waves directed into the tissues*
Ultravate / *cream* / *topical corticosteroid anti-inflammatory* / D
umbilicus / the navel
-um / *noun ending* / e.g., calci**um**
Unasyn / *penicillin-type antibiotic* / *for pneumonia* / D
uncinate / *shaped like a hook*
Ungerleider / *x-ray technique*
ungual / *nails*
ungualabia / *edges of nails*
unguium
uni- *one*
Uni-Decon / *decongestant* / *antihistamine* / D
Uni-Dur / theophylline / once daily antiasthmatic / bronchodilator / D
unilateral / *affecting one side only*
Uniphyl / theophylline / *bronchodilator* / D
Univasc / *antihypertensive* / *ACE inhibitor* / D
Unna boot / Unna paste boot / *bandage*

Additional Entries

____

____

____

____

unresectable
upper pole of kidney
UPT / urine pregnancy test
uptake / *absorption and incorporation of a substance by living tissue* / e.g., iodine by the thyroid gland
Ur / UR / *urine* / *urinary*
urachal cancer (Uro) / *type of bladder cancer*
urate / *a uric acid salt*
-ure / *result of an action, device* / e.g., expos**ure**, press**ure**
ure-, urea-, ureo-, uria- / *urea* / *urine*
urea kinetics
urea nitrogen
urease / *an enzyme* / *used in clinical assays of plasma urea concentrations*
URF / uterine relaxing factor
Urecholine / bethanechol chloride / *postsurgical cholinergic bladder muscle stimulant* / D
urelcosis / *ulceration of the urinary tract*
uremia/-ic / *excessive urea and other nitrogenous waste in blood*
ureteral (Uro) / *pertaining to the ureter, the tube that carries urine to the bladder*
ureteral bowel syndrome (Uro)
ureteral lithiasis / *calculi in the ureter* / *stone(s) in the ureter*
ureterectasia (Uro) / *ureter dilation*
ureteroneocystostomy / ureterocystostomy (Uro) / *surgical implantation of ureter into bladder*
ureteropelvic (Uro) / *pertaining to the ureter and the pelvis*
ureth-, urethr-, urethro- / *the urethra*
urethritis (Uro) / *inflammation of the urethra*
urethrotrigonitis / *inflammation of the urethra and trigone of the bladder*

Additional Entries

urethrovesical / *pertaining to the urethra and the bladder*

URI / upper respiratory infection

uri-, uric-, urico- / *uric acid*

-uria / urine

uricemia / *excess uric acid or urates in the blood* / gout

uricosurics / *agents that promote excretion of uric acid in the urine*

Urimar-T / *urinary anti-infective / antiseptic / analgesic / antispasmodic*

urinalysis showed trace protein

urine for 5HIAA

urine grew out

urine micral / T

urine oxalate

urine tandem icon

Urised / *urinary anti-infective / analgesic / antispasmodic / acidifier* / D

Urispas / flavoxate / *urinary antispasmodic* / D

urobilin / *brown pigment formed by the oxidation of urobilinogen / may form in stools or urine after exposure to air*

urobilinogen / *decomposition product of bilirubin / precursor of urobilin*

Urocit-K / potassium citrate / *urinary alkalizer / nephrolithiasis preventative* / D

urolithiasis (Uro) / *calculi or stone(s) in the urinary tract*

uropathy (Uro) / *any disorder of the urinary tract*

uroporphyrin synthetase (Uro)

URQ / upper right quadrant (abdomen)

USO / unilateral salpingo-oophorectomy

urosepsis (Uro) / *invasion of microorganisms from the urinary tract into the bloodstream*

Additional Entries

ursodeoxycholic acid / ursodiol / Actigall / *dissolves gallstones* / D
ursodiol / Actigall / *anticholelithogenic* / D
urticaria (Derm) / *itching skin* / *itching wheals*
uterovesical (Gyn) / *pertaining to the uterus and the bladder*
UTI / urinary tract infection
uveitis/-es (Oph) / *inflammation of the uveal tract*
UVJ obstruction (GU) / ureterovesical junction (obstruction)
uvula / *small, fleshy body projecting downward from the middle of the soft palate*
uvulectomy / *surgical removal of the uvula*
UW / unilateral weakness

Additional Entries

____

____

____

____

vacuole / *a small space in any tissue*
vacuolization phenomena / *the process of forming vacuoles*
vacuum joint phenomenon
vagin-, vagino- / *the vagina*
vagina (Gyn) / *female genital canal*
vaginismus (Gyn) / *painful spasm of vagina*
vaginitis / *inflammation of the vagina*
vaginosis / *any disease of the vagina* / e.g., bacterial v.
Vagisil / *topical local anesthetic* / *antipruritic* / *anti-fungal* / D [OTC]
vagotomy / *interruption of vagus nerve impulses* / *division of the vagus nerve*
Val / evaluation
valgus / *bent outward* / *deformity in which angulation is away from the midline of the body*
Valisone / betamethasone / *cream* / *topical corticosteroid* / D
Valium / diazepam / *sedative* / *anxiolytic* / *skeletal muscle relaxant* / *anticonvulsant adjunct* / D
vallecula / *furrow*
valproic acid / Depakene / Depakote / *anticonvulsant* / D
Valsalva maneuver / *any forced expiratory effort against a closed airway* / *attempt to forcibly exhale with the glottis, nose, or mouth closed* / *used to study cardiovascular effects*
Valtrex / valacyclovir / *for herpes* / D
valvular / *pertaining to a valve*
Van Buren sound
Vancenase / *intranasal steroidal anti-inflammatory* / D
Vanceril inhaler / *corticosteroid* / *for bronchial asthma* / D
vancomycin / Lyphocin / Vancocin / Vancoled / *glycopeptide bactericidal antibiotic* / D
Vantin / cefpodoxime proxetil / *cephalosporin-type antibiotic* / D

Additional Entries

variceal / varix / *vein*

varicella / *acute contagious disease*

varices / *plural of varix*

varicocele / *condition characterized by abnormal dilation of veins in the spermatic cord*

variegated / *varied in color or appearance / marked with patches or spots of varying colors*

Varilux (Oph) / *eyeglass lens*

Varivax / *chicken pox vaccine*

varus / *bent inward*

vas-, vaso-, vasculo- / *blood vessel / duct / canal that carries fluid*

vasa vasorum / *small arteries*

vascularization / *formation of new blood vessels*

vasculature / *vascular network of an organ or body area*

vasculitis / angiitis / *inflammation of a blood vessel*

vas deferens / *duct that carries sperm from the epididymis to the penis*

Vaseretic / enalapril maleate / *antihypertensive* / D

Vasocon-A (Oph) / naphazoline / *eye drops / topical ocular decongestant / vasoconstrictor* / D [OTC]

vasodepression / *relaxed blood vessels with vasodilation, causing lowered blood pressure*

vasodepressor syncope

Vasodilan / isoxsuprine / *peripheral vasodilator* / D

vasoganglion / *mass of blood vessels*

vasomotor / *pertaining to dilation or constriction of blood vessels*

vasospasm/-tic / *contraction or hypertonia of blood vessels*

Vasosulf (Oph) / *ophthalmic bacteriostatic / decongestant* / D

Vasotec / enalapril / *antihypertensive / ACE inhibitor* / D

vasovagal / *pertaining to action of the vagus nerve upon blood vessels*

Additional Entries

---

vastus / *great* / *pertaining to muscles* / e.g., v. lateralis; v. medialis

Vater papilla / duodeni major / *duodenal end of drainage systems of pancreatic and common bile ducts*

V-Cillin K / penicillin V potassium / *bactericidal antibiotic* / D

VD / venereal disease

vectorcardiography/-gram (Cardio) / *electronic procedure in which heart activity is represented by vector loops*

Veetids / penicillin V potassium / *bactericidal antibiotic* / D

Veillonella / *microorganisms*

Velban / vinblastine sulfate / *antineoplastic* / *for lung, breast, and testicular cancers* / D

velcro rales / *lung sounds like Velcro being torn apart*

velopharyngeal / *referring to the soft palate and the posterior nasopharyngeal wall*

Velpeau deformity / *peculiar deformity seen in Colles fracture*

vena-, vene-, veno- / *veins* / *venous*

vena cava / *vessel that conveys blood toward the heart, or from the heart to the right atrium*

Venalot depot

venipuncture / *puncture of a vein*

venisection / phlebotomy

venlafaxine / Effexor / *antidepressant* / D

venoclysis / phleboclysis / *washing out* / *intravenous injection of a fluid in quantity*

venogram V

venostasis / *abnormally slow flow of blood in veins*

venous hyperemia / venosity / *excess venous blood in a part*

venous lake

venous stasis changes

Ventolin / Proventil / Volmax / albuterol / *bronchodilator* / D

Additional Entries

ventilatory failure / *failure to control pulmonary ventilation*
ventral / *the belly* / *anterior* / *undersurface*
ventric-, ventriculo- / *ventricle*
ventricle / *normal body cavity* / e.g., cerebral v.; v. of heart; laryngeal v.
ventricular / *pertaining to a ventricle*
ventriculogram (Cardio)
ventriculotomy / *surgical incision into a ventricle*
ventrogluteal / *muscle*
verapamil (Cardio) / *sustained release medication* / *coronary vasodilator* / *calcium channel blocker* / D
Verelan / verapamil / *antihypertensive* / *calcium channel blocker* / D
Vermox / mebendazole / *anthelmintic* / *for pinworms* / D
vernix / e.g., v. caseosa / *fatty substance and sebaceous matter that covers the skin of the fetus*
verruca/-ae (Derm) / wart / *horny-surfaced growth*
   v. acuminata / *moist wart about the genitals and the anus*
   v. vulgaris / *common warts* / *usually on hands and fingers*
verruciform / *shaped like or resembling a wart*
verrucous / verrucose / *rough* / *warty*
Versed / midazolam / *for injection* / *general anesthesia adjunct* / D
versicolor / *variegated* / *many-colored*
vertebral bodies / *of or pertaining to a vertebra*
vertex / (pl.) vertices / *scalp* / *top of skull*
vertebrobasilar / *disease involving vertebral and basilar arteries*
vertiginous / *dizzy* / *experiencing vertigo*
vertigo / *dizzy feeling* / *sensation of spinning or whirling motion*
verumontanum (Uro) / *part of the urethral crest*
vesicle / *bladder* / *small sac containing liquid or gas*
vesicoureteral (Uro) / *pertaining to the bladder and the ureters*
vesicular / *small saclike bodies*

Additional Entries

____

____

____

____

vesiculation / *presence of vesicles*
vesiculopapular / *vesicles and papules* / *papules increasing in size due to fluid intake*
vesnarinone (Cardio) / *drug study*
vestibular test
Vexol (Oph) / rimexolone / *eye drops* / *ophthalmic topical corticosteroidal anti-inflammatory* / D
VHDL / very-high-density lipoprotein
Vibramycin / doxycycline / *tetracycline-type antibiotic* / D
Vibra-Tabs / doxycycline / D
vibratory / *vibrating* / *causing vibration*
Vibrio parahaemolyticus / *bacteria*
Vicodin / hydrocodone and acetaminophen / *narcotic analgesic* / D
Vicon-C / vitamin B complex with vitamin C / D [OTC]
vicryl sutures
villoglandular
villonodular synovitis / *pigmented*
villose / villous / *covered with villi* / *shaggy*
villus / *protrusion* / *projection from the surface*
vincristine / *antineoplastic* / D
Vioform / clioquinol / *topical antifungal* / *antibacterial* / D
Viokase / pancrelipase / *digestive enzymes* / *for pancreatic insufficiency* / D
violaceous / *violet or purple discoloration, usually of skin*
Virchow angle / *angle between nasobasilar line and nasosubnasal line*
viremia / *virus malaise*
viridans Streptococci / *former name for alpha-hemolytic streptococci*
virologist / *microbiologist specializing in virology*

Additional Entries

Viscoheel cushion
VisCo Soles / *in shoes*
viscera / *plural of viscus* / *organs in the cavities of the body*
visceromegaly / *abnormal enlargement of viscera*
visceroptosis/-ia / *movement of viscera from normal positions*
viscosity / *fluid state that resists flowing*
viscous / *sticky* / *thick*
Viscous Xylocaine / *gargle*
viscus / *singular of viscera*
Vistaril / hydroxyzine / *anxiolytic* / D
Vitallium / *surgical alloy*
vitiligo (Derm) / *skin disease*
vitreous (Oph) / *glassy* / *glasslike*
Vitron-C / *iron* / *hematinic* / D
Vivactil / protriptyline / *tricyclic antidepressant* / D
Vivarin / *stimulant* / *analeptic* / D [OTC]
VLDL / very-low-density lipoprotein
vocal cord
volar / *palm of hand* / *sole of foot*
volar wrist flexion crease
Volkmann contracture (Ortho) / *after severe injury of the elbow joint, contracture of the fingers and wrist with loss of power*
Volmax / albuterol / *bronchodilator* / D
Voltaren / diclofenac / *nonsteroidal anti-inflammatory* / *anti-arthritic* / *analgesic* / D
volvulus / *intestinal obstruction*
vomer / *nasal septum*
von Gierke disease / *glycogen storage disease*
von Recklinghausen disease / neurofibromatosis / *tumors of various sizes on peripheral nerves*
vonWillebrand disease / *congenital hemorrhagic diathesis*

Additional Entries

VoSol / acetic acid (Oto) / *otic solution* / D
Votox / *for dystonia retrocollis* / D
VPB (Cardio) / ventricular premature beat
vp-16 / etoposide / D
V/Q scan / *ventilation* / *perfusion study*
vulvovaginitis (Ob-Gyn) / *inflammation of vulva and
    vagina*
V-tach (Cardio) / ventricular tachycardia

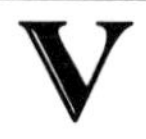

Additional Entries

Waardenburg syndrome / *congenital defect* / *an autosomal dominant disorder with white forelock, white eyelashes, leukoderma, and sometimes, deafness*

Wagner Grade I / *ulceration*

Waldenstrom macroglobulinemia

Waldeyer ring / *ring of tonsillar tissue that encircles the nasopharynx and oropharynx* / *formed by lingual, pharyngeal and faucial tonsils*

Waldryl / Walgreen's generic Benadryl

Walker syndrome *(see Dandy-Walker)*

Walthard islets or inclusions (Gyn)/ *germinal epithelium of ovary*

Wangensteen tube / *nose to stomach tube for suction to maintain decompression*

warfarin / Coumadin / *anticoagulant* / D

warehousemen's itch (Derm) / *eczema of hands from handling irritating substances*

Warm and Form / *corset*

water brash / *heartburn, with regurgitation of sour fluid into mouth*

water intoxication / *excess water and sodium retention*

Waterhouse-Friderichsen syndrome / *malignant epidemic cerebrospinal meningitis*

Waters view / *x-ray of sinuses*

Waterston shunt / *connection between ascending aorta and right pulmonary artery* / *to relieve pulmonary stenosis*

WBC / white blood cell / white blood count

WDWN / well developed, well nourished

Weber-Christian disease / *panniculitis* / *inflammation of subcutaneous fat*

Weber test (Otology)

weird

Additional Entries

____

____

____

____

Wegener granulomatosis / *condition characterized by the forma-
tion of inflammatory cells / lesions of entire respiratory tract,
and glomerulonephritis*
Wellbutrin / *for smoking cessation / for ADD* / D
Wenckebach arrhythmia (Cardio)
Werdnig-Hoffman paralysis
Wernicke encephalopathy (Neuro)
Wertheim operation / *radical hysterectomy for carcinoma of uterus*
Westcort / *cream / topical corticosteroid*
Westergren method / *sedimentation rate* / T
Western Blot / T
Wharton duct / *duct of the submandibular salivary gland*
whiff (Cardio) / *sound in the heart*
Whipple operation / *removal of the distal third of the stomach,
entire duodenum, and head of the pancreas*
Whitman operation (Ortho) / *arthroplasty of the hip joint*
whorle / *spiral turn, as a turn of the cochlea of the inner ear*
Wigraine / *suppositories / migraine-specific vasoconstrictor* / D
Williams flexion / *exercise*
Willis antrum / *pertaining to the pyloric part of the stomach*
Wilms tumor / *malignant tumor of the kidneys in children*
WNF / well-nourished female
WNL / within normal limits
WNM / well-nourished male
Wood's light / Wood's rays / *ultraviolet rays / used to detect
fluorescent materials in skin and hair in certain diseases* /
e.g., in tinea capitis
wormian bones / ossa suturalia / *small, irregular bones in the
cranial sutures*
WPW / Wolff-Parkinson-White (syndrome)
Wright peak flow (Pulm)

Additional Entries

____

____

____

____

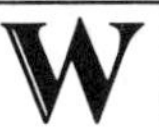

wristlets
wrote memory / wrote fashion...**NO!** (see "rote fashion")
Wuchereria / bancrofti / malayi / *roundworms*
Wycillin IM / penicillin G procaine / *bactericidal antibiotic* / D
Wygesic / propoxyphene and acetaminophen / *narcotic analgesic* / D
Wytensin / guanabenz acetate / *antihypertensive* / D

Additional Entries

Xanax / alprazolam / *anxiolytic* / D
xanth-, xantho- / *yellow* / *yellowish*
xanthelasma/-asmata / *yellow spots on eyelids*
xanthene / xanthine / *a product of oxidation*
xanthinuria / *abnormally large amounts of xanthene in urine*
xanthofibroma thecocellulare / dermatofibroma
xanthochromia / *yellow patches in the skin*
xanthoma / *yellow nodule*
Xenical / *drug study* / *antiobesity agent* / D
xeno- / *strange* / *foreign*
xenon arc / *gaseous element* / *atomic number 54*
Xeroform / *gauze*
xerosis / *abnormal dryness*
xerostomia / *dry mouth*
xiphoidalgia
xiphoid / *shaped like a sword*
xiphoid process / *distal end of sternum*
Xi-scan / *type of x-ray*
xylene / xylol / *mixture of isometric hydrocarbons used in making lacquers and rubber cement*
Xylocaine / *injectable local anesthetic* / D

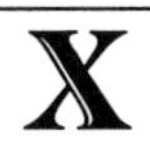

Additional Entries

257

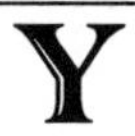

-y / *result of an action* / *inquiry* / *a condition* /
  e.g., dreamy
YAG / *yttrium, argon, garnet* (laser) / *laser surgery*
Yersinia / *bacteria*
yersiniosis / *infectious disease*
Yocon / *sympatholytic* / *aphrodisiac* / D
yohimbine / Aphrodyne / Yohimex / *for impotence* /
  claimed to be an aphrodisiac / D

<hr>

Additional Entries

____

____

____

____

Zantac / *gastric and duodenal ulcer treatment* / D
Zaroxolyn / metolazone / *diuretic* / *antihypertensive* / D
Z-Bec / *vitamin* / *zinc supplement* / D
Zeasorb / miconazole / *powder* / *absorbent* / D [OTC]
Zemuron / rocuronium bromide / *neuromuscular blocking agent for anesthesia* / D
Zenker fixative
Zestoretic / *antihypertensive* / D
Zestril / lisinopril / *antihypertensive* / *ACE inhibitor* / D
Ziac / *antihypertensive* / D
Zincon / pyrithione zinc / *shampoo* / *antiseborrheic* / *antibacterial* / D [OTC]
Zithromax / Z-Pak / azithromycin / *macrolide antibiotic* / D
Zocor / simvastatin / *cholesterol-lowering antihyperlipidemic* / D
Zoladex / goserelin acetate / *palliative hormonal chemotherapy* / *for prostatic carcinoma, breast cancer, and endometriosis* / D
Zollinger-Ellison syndrome (Gastro) / *triad: 1) atypical peptic ulcers, 2) extreme gastric hyperacidity, and 3) tumors of the pancreas or duodenum*
Zoloft /sertraline hydrochloride / *antidepressant* / D
Zomax / D
Zonalon / doxepin / *cream* / *topical antihistamine* / *antipruritic* / D
ZORprin / aspirin / D
zosteriform / zosteroid / *resembling herpes zoster*
Zostrix / capsaicin / *topical analgesic* / D
Zovirax / acyclovir / *antiviral* / *for herpes infections* / D
Z-Pak / Zithromax / *macrolide antibiotic* / D
Z-plasty / *to relax contractures*
ZSB / zero stool (since) birth
Zyflo / *for asthma* / D
zygapophysis (Ortho) / *vertebra*

Additional Entries

____

____

____

____

Zyloprim / allopurinol / *investigation antineoplastic* / D
zymosan / *a carbohydrate*
Zyrtec / cetirizine / *once-daily antihistamine* / D

Additional Entries

NOTES

ABOUT RAYVE PRODUCTIONS

Rayve Productions is an award-winning small publisher of books and music. Current publications are primarily in the following categories:

> (1) Business guidebooks for home-based businesses and other entrepreneurs
> (2) Quality children's books and music
> (3) History books about America and her regions, and an heirloom-quality journal for creating personal histories.

Rayve Productions' mail-order catalog offers the above items plus business books, software, music, and other enjoyable items produced by others.

Our eclectic collection of business resources and gift items has something to please everyone.

A FREE catalog is available upon request.

Come visit us at www.spannet.org/rayve.

BUSINESS & CAREER

☆ *Smart Tax Write-offs: Hundreds of tax deduction ideas for home-based businesses, independent contractors, all entrepreneurs*
by Norm Ray, CPA

ISBN 1-877810-20-7, softcover, $12.95, 1996 pub.

Fun-to-read, easy-to-use guidebook that encourages entrepreneurs to be aggressive and creative in taking legitimate tax deductions. Includes valuable checklist of over 600 write-off ideas. Every small business owner's "must read." (Recommended by *Home Office Computing, Small Business Opportunities, Spare Time, Independent Business Magazine*).

☆ *The Independent Medical Transcriptionist, 3rd edition: The comprehensive guidebook for career success in a home-based medical transcription business*   by Donna Avila-Weil, CMT and Mary Glaccum, CMT

ISBN 1-877810-23-1, softcover, $34.95, 1997 pub.

The industry's premier reference book for medical transcription entrepreneurs. (Recommended by *Journal of the American Association for Medical Transcription, Entrepreneur, Small Business Opportunities)*

☆ *Independent Medical Coding: The comprehensive guidebook for career success as a home-based medical coder*
by Donna Avila-Weil, CMT and Rhonda Regan, CCS

ISBN 1-877810-17-7, softcover, $34.95, 1997 pub.

How to start and successfully run your own professional independent medical coding business. Step-by-step instructions.

☆ *Easy Financials for Your Home-based Business*   by Norm Ray, CPA

ISBN 1-877810-92-4, softcover, $19.95, 1992 pub.

Small business & home-based business expert helps you save time by making your work easier, and save money by nailing down your tax deductions.
(Recommended by *Wilson Library Bulletin, The Business Journal, National Home Business Report)*

☆ *Internal Medicine Words*   by Minta Danna

ISBN 1-877810-68-1, softcover, $29.95, 1997 pub.

Over 8,000 words and terms related to internal medicine. A valuable spelling and terminology usage resource for medical transcriptionists, medical writers and editors, court reporters, medical records personnel, and others working with medical documentation.

☆ *Shrinking the Globe into Your Company's Hands: The step-by-step international trade guide for small businesses*   by Sidney R. Lawrence, PE

ISBN 1-877810-46-0, softcover, $24.95, 1997 pub.

An expert in foreign trade shows U.S. small business owners how to market and export products and services safely and profitably.

HISTORY

☆ *20 Tales of California: A rare collection of western stories* by Hector Lee
ISBN 1-877810-63-0, hardcover, $16.95
ISBN 1-877810-62-2, softcover, $9.95, 1997 pub.
Mysterious and romantic tales: real life and folklore set in various California locations. Includes ideas for family outings and classroom field trips.

☆ *Link Across America: A story of the historic Lincoln Highway* — see Children's Books

☆ *Windsor, The Birth of a City*　　　　　by Gabriel A. Fraire
ISBN 1-877810-91-6, hardcover, $21.95, 1991 pub.
Fascinating case study of political and social issues surrounding city incorporation of Windsor, California, 1978—1991. LAFCO impact.

☆ *LifeTimes, The Life Experiences Journal*
ISBN 1-877810-34-7, hardcover, $49.95
World's easiest, most fun and useful personal journal. Handsome heirloom quality with gilt-edged pages. Over 150 information categories to record your life experiences. Winner of national award for excellence.

GENERAL

☆ *Nancy's Candy Cookbook: How to make candy at home the easy way*
by Nancy Shipman
ISBN 1-877810-65-7, softcover, $14.95, 1996 pub.
Have fun and save money by making candy at home at a fraction of candy store prices. More than 100 excellent candy recipes — from Grandma's delicious old-fashioned fudge to modern gourmet truffles. Includes many children's favorites, too.

☆ *Joy of Reading: One family's fun-filled guide to reading success*
by Debbie Duncan
ISBN 1-877810-45-2, softcover, $14.95, 1998 pub.
A dynamic author and mother, and an expert on children's literature, shares her family's personal reading success stories. You'll be inspired and entertained by this lighthearted, candid glimpse into one family's daily experiences as they cope with the ups and downs of life. Through it all, there is love, and an abundance of wonderful books to mark the milestones along the way.

CHILDREN'S BOOKS & MUSIC

☆ *Link Across America: A story of the historic Lincoln Highway*
by Mary Elizabeth Anderson

ISBN 1-877810-97-5, hardcover, $14.95, 1997 pub.

It began with a long-ago dream . . . a road that would run clear across America! The dream became reality in 1914 as the Lincoln Highway began to take form, to eventually run from New York City to San Francisco. Venture from past to present experiencing transportation history. Topics include Abraham Lincoln, teams of horses, seedling miles, small towns, making concrete, auto courts, Burma Shave signs, classic cars and road rallies. Color photos along today's Lincoln Highway remnants, b/w historical photos, map and list of cities along the old Lincoln Highway. (Ages 7-13 & their parents, grandparents & great-grandparents)

☆ *The Perfect Orange: A tale from Ethiopia*
by Frank P. Araujo, PhD; illustrated by Xiao Jun Li

ISBN 1-877810-94-0, hardcover, $16.95, 1994 pub., Toucan Tales volume 2

Inspiring gentle folktale. Breathtaking watercolors dramatize ancient Ethiopia's contrasting pastoral charm and majesty. Illustrations are rich with Ethiopian details. Story reinforces values of generosity and selflessness over greed and self-centeredness. Glossary of Ethiopian terms and pronunciation key.

(**PBS** *Storytime* **Selection**; Recommended by *School Library Journal, Faces, MultiCultural Review, Small Press Magazine, The Five Owls, Wilson Library Bulletin)*

☆ *Nekane, the Lamiña & the Bear: A tale of the Basque Pyrenees*
by Frank P. Araujo, PhD; illustrated by Xiao Jun Li

ISBN 1-877810-01-0, hardcover, $16.95, 1993 pub., Toucan Tales volume 1

Delightful Basque folktale pits appealing, quick-witted young heroine against mysterious villain. Lively, imaginative narrative, sprinkled with Basque phrases. Vibrant watercolor images. Glossary of Basque terms and pronunciation key.

(Recommended by School Library Journal, Publishers Weekly, Kirkus Reviews, Booklist, Wilson Library Bulletin, The Basque Studies Program Newsletter: University of Nevada, BCCB, The Five Owls)

☆ *The Laughing River: A folktale for peace*
by Elizabeth Haze Vega; illustrated by Ashley Smith, 1995 pub.

ISBN 1-877810-35-5   hardcover book, $16.95

ISBN 1-877810-36-3   companion musical audiotape, $9.95

ISBN 1-877810-37-1   book & musical audiotape combo, $23.95

Drum kit, $9.95

Book, musical audiotape & drum kit combo, $29.95

Two fanciful African tribes are in conflict until the laughing river bubbles melodiously into their lives, bringing fun, friendship, peace. Lyrical fanciful folktale of conflict resolution. Mesmerizing music. Dancing, singing and drumming instructions. Orff approach. (Recommended by *School Library Journal)*

☆ *When Molly Was in the Hospital: A book for brothers and sisters of hospitalized children*

by Debbie Duncan; illustrated by Nina Ollikainen, MD
ISBN 1-877810-44-4, hardcover, $12.95, 1994 pub.
Anna's little sister, Molly, has been very ill and had to have an operation. Anna tells us all about the experience from her point of view. Sensitive, insightful, heartwarming story. A support and comfort for siblings and those who love them. Authentic. Realistic. Effective.
(Winner of 1995 Benjamin Franklin Award: Best Children's Picture Book. Recommended by *Children's Book Insider, School Library Journal, Disabilities Resources Monthly*)

☆ *Night Sounds*

by Lois G. Grambling; illustrated by Randall F. Ray
ISBN 1-877810-77-0, hardcover, $12.95   ISBN 1-877810-83-5, softcover, $6.95, 1996 pub.
Perfect bedtime story. Ever so gently, a child's thoughts slip farther and farther away, moving from purring cat at bedside and comical creatures in the yard to distant trains and church bells, and then at last, to sleep. Imaginative, lilting text and daringly unpretentious b/w watercolor illustrations

☆ *Los Sonidos de la Noche*

by Lois G. Grambling; illustrated by Randall F. Ray
(Spanish edition of *Night Sounds*), 1996 pub.
ISBN 1-877810-76-2, hardcover, $12.95   ISBN 1-877810-82-7, softcover, $6.95

ORDER

For mail orders please complete this order form and forward with check, money order or credit card information to Rayve Productions, POB 726, Windsor CA 95492. If paying with a credit card, you can fax this completed form to Rayve Productions at 707.838.2220.

You can also order at our web site at www.spannet.org/rayve.

☐ Please send me the following book(s):

Title _______________________ Price _________ Qty _____ Amount _________

Title _______________________ Price _________ Qty _____ Amount _________

Title _______________________ Price _________ Qty _____ Amount _________

Title _______________________ Price _________ Qty _____ Amount _________

Total Amount _________

Sales Tax: Californians please add 7.5% sales tax   Sales Tax _________

S/H: Book rate --- $3 for first book + $.50 each additional   Shipping _________

Priority --- $4 for first book + $.75 each additional

Total _________

Name _______________________   Phone _________

Address _______________________

City State Zip _______________________

☐ Check enclosed $ _______________________   Date _________

☐ Charge my Visa/MC/Discover/AMEX $ _______________________

Credit card # _______________________   Exp. _________

Signature _______________________   *Thank you!*